THE
TUIN

COMHAIRLE CHONTAE ÁTHA CLIATH THEAS
SOUTH DUBLIN COUNTY LIBRARIES

STEWARTS HOSPITAL BRANCH
TO RENEW ANY ITEM TEL:

Items should be returned on or before the last date below. Fines, as displayed in the Library, will be charged on overdue items.

THE THIN
COMMANDMENTS

The **TEN** no-fail diet strategies of the winners at weight control

Dr Stephen Gullo

RODALE

This edition first published in 2005 by
Rodale International Ltd
7–10 Chandos Street
London
W1G 9AD
www.rodale.co.uk

Printed and bound in the UK by CPI Bath using acid-free paper from sustainable sources.
1 3 5 7 9 8 6 4 2

A CIP record for this book is available from the British Library

ISBN 1-4050-7753-0

This paperback edition distributed to the book trade by Pan Macmillan Ltd

Notice
This book is intended as a reference volume only, not as a medical manual. The information given here is designed to help you make informed decisions about your health. It is not intended as a substitute for any treatment that may have been prescribed by your doctor. If you suspect that you have a medical problem, we urge you to seek competent medical help.

Mention of specific companies, organizations or authorities in this book does not imply endorsement by the publisher, nor does mention of specific companies, organizations or authorities in the book imply that they endorse it. Internet addresses and telephone numbers given in this book were accurate at the time it went to press.

To Ruth Edelman

Indomitable advocate on behalf of mental health and humanitarian causes across America, leader in the civic life of the city of Chicago, who, along with her daughter, Renee Edelman, has been the greatest of friends and advisors. Thank you for being a true 'guardian angel'.

To Dr Austin Kutscher

Distinguished professor in the department of psychiatry at Columbia University and president of the American Institute of Life-Threatening Illness at the Columbia-Presbyterian Medical Center, who has been my most inspiring teacher and mentor. Your pioneering work and monumental contributions to the sciences and health care have touched the lives of thousands and have profoundly shaped my professional life and all that I have done and will do in my career. I am forever grateful.

To my colleagues in nutrition, bariatric medicine and dietetics

Who work each day on the front lines of weight control and who have contributed so much to the management of obesity and weight problems.

Contents

Acknowledgements

Many people have nurtured both my life and work, and I will always be grateful to them.

My family has loved and supported me unconditionally, and to my sisters, Angela Barna, Marianne Froelich and Antoinette Pahlck; my nephews and nieces Christian and Karen Hanny and now little Kate Rose Hanny, Matthew Touron and Maurene Levine; and my brothers-in-law, Joseph Barna, Allan Froelich and Robert Pahlck, I say a profound *thank you*. I will always owe a special debt of gratitude to my sister Angela and my brother-in-law Joseph, who cared for my father so selflessly during his final illness.

I have been blessed with a loving second family in Mathew and Lee Love, along with Wendy and Lance Barnard and the late and beloved Florence Lazar-Galleau, who generously donated so much of her time and talents to help me as I started my career.

Along the road of my life, many friends have made enormous contributions to my growth: Dr David and the late Marilyn Kohn, Drs Daniel and Justine Carr, Duane Perez, Jason Capuano, Gloria Futterweit, Dr Dan Cherico, Dr Marc Shatz, Dr Henry Berger, Anthony Abreu, Peter Swersey, John Contini, Anne Hearst, George Paxinos, Steve Zubkoff, Kent Keets, Douglas Kohn, Ronni Janoff-Weinstein and Barry Weinstein, Scott Yacker, Erica Morales, Dee Kerner, Mike Nelligan, Joanna Silverblatt, Luis Soto, and, of course, my dear friends and associates Edoardo Danilan and Nina Danilan. I am particularly grateful for the personal and professional support given to me and my work by my esteemed friends Jack Rudin, Leon Wagener, Gloria Milstein Flanzer and Louis Flanzer. The rarest of human qualities is generosity of spirit and they are the definition of this spirit.

All that I have and will accomplish in my professional life would not be possible without the support of a gifted and dedicated team that assists me each day at the Institute for Health & Weight Sciences. Rosemarie Passaro has been with me from the very beginning, as a colleague and cherished friend, and her stewardship of our financial matters is so crucial. I will always be grateful to a remarkable man, her late husband, Tom Passaro. Norbert Bogner, my office manager and friend, oversees the daily operations and deals brilliantly with my often crazy schedule. Mike Nelligan is our 'troubleshooter'. He 'makes it all happen'. Mikhail Pomeranets skilfully assisted me with numerous aspects of this book and gave me and my writers invaluable guidance on computer matters.

At crucial points in my development, I was able to call on the wisdom of several professors and advisors who enhanced my life with their guidance: Dr Rosalea Schonbar, late director of the clinical psychology programme at Columbia University, Dr David Peretz, the late Dr B. Schoenberg and Revd Harold Robertson.

Two of my closest friends, Dr Andrew Lassman and Lenin De La Cruz, have been constant sources of support and encouragement to me at each step in the writing of this book. Andrew is also a brilliant young scientist who gives me a forum to share and formulate scientific ideas. I thank both of them in these pages so they will know how much their support has meant to me. A top personal trainer and colleague, Brett Austin, contributed his scientific knowledge and insights to evaluating important research along with introducing me to the concept of volumizing.

Each week I call on the professional expertise of a group of gifted advisors: Dr David Kohn, Hon. Michael Kalnick and Nellon Chu. Their guidance has enabled me to navigate around so many of life's pitfalls. I also want to add a special word of thanks to a singularly talented litigator, Alan Green.

Miriam Rubin, a gifted, world-class chef, provided invaluable assistance with recipes and cooking skills, and Elissa Meadow, CEO and proprietor of Los Angeles's new Solar Harvest restaurant, was extraordinarily generous in contributing some of that restaurant's outstanding recipes.

Luis Soto, one of New York's premier trainers and life coaches, has helped many of my clients achieve their optimal potential and has been a wise and gifted advisor on exercise.

In recent years a number of outstanding people have entered my life and shared their friendship and expertise with me. Renee Edelman has always also been so generous with her time and expertise, and the success of *Thin Tastes Better* would never have been possible without Renee and her mother, Ruth Edelman. I also want to thank a brilliant journalist, George Christy, for his support. Both his pen and his intellect are a true gift to so many.

In the writing and marketing of this book, so many individuals gave invaluable guidance. Holly McCord, former nutrition editor at *Prevention* magazine, initially suggested to me that I bring this book to Rodale. Tami Booth, vice president, editor-in-chief of women's health books at Rodale, was the first person in publishing to read the proposal for this book and her appreciation for my work was a determining factor in selecting Rodale as my publisher. Tami introduced me to the team that would shape this work. Margot Schupf, executive editor, has guided me throughout the writing of this book with her insights and wisdom. Whenever I had a question or concern, Margot has always been there for me. Editor Christine Bucks has laboured endlessly to edit this book and articulate its message. I am grateful for her important work, most of all her patience through all of my rewrites. I have found in the executive and professional staffs of Rodale gifted leaders and individuals who have supported and shaped this book: Amy Rhodes, vice president and publisher of trade books; Nancy Bailey, senior project editor; Cathy Gruhn, director of publicity, trade books; Cindy Ratzlaff, vice president of Rodale books; Dana Bacher, marketing director of trade books; Leslie Schneider, director of trade sales; and Sara Sellar, editorial assistant, women's health books, all of whom have been enormously helpful with their professional excellence. In a very real sense, I owe a unique debt to the Rodale family, for it was as a young boy reading *Prevention* magazine that my interest in health and health care first began.

I want to thank the prominent researchers and scientists whose pioneering work has been discussed in this book and who generously agreed to be interviewed: Dr Virend K. Somers, professor of medicine in the division of cardiovascular disease and hypertension at the Mayo Clinic School of Medicine; Richard A. Anderson, PhD, lead scientist at the Beltsville Human Nutrition Research Center in Maryland; Michael Zemel, PhD, chairman of the nutrition department at the University of Tennessee; Dr Sarah Leibowitz, professor at the Rockefeller University laboratory of behavioural neuroscience in New York City; C. Wayne Calloway, endocrinologist at George Washington University in Washington, D.C.; Linda Bartoshuk, professor of the Yale University School of Medicine; Valerie Duffy, PhD, assistant professor of dietetics at the University of Connecticut; and Dr Walter Futterweit, clinical professor of medicine at Mount Sinai Medical School and chief, endocrine clinics, at Mt. Sinai – one of the nation's premier endocrinologists. Dr Futterweit first introduced me to Polycystic Ovarian Syndrome and generously helped me to understand its implications for weight management. He is truly the consummate 'doctors' doctor' and a great healer.

Robert Barnett, Esq., of Williams & Connolly, was the erudite and gifted attorney who made possible the sale of this book and who once again proved the wisdom of our mutual friends, Ruth and Daniel Edelman. I want to also thank Sylvia, Mr Barnett's executive assistant, who 'always gets it right'.

No acknowledgements would be complete without thanking a great friend and author, Sugar Rautbord. Through her unmatched abilities to persuade and her honoured position in the media community, she played a decisive role in the success of *Thin Tastes Better*. I will always be in her debt. Thank you, Sugar. You are the very best.

Carol Southern of Crown/Carol Southern Books was the gifted editor of my earlier work, *Thin Tastes Better*. That book would never have become a reality without her vision and support. The fact that it went on to become a national bestseller is a tribute to her leadership. Catherine Heusel-Grillo and Joseph Amodio were the most talented writers who made *Thin Tastes Better* possible. Catherine has become a friend I cherish deeply. It was she who crafted the organization and the writing of the proposal for this present book. She did so much to brilliantly take this book from concept to reality.

A team of gifted writers shaped this book and brought it to you. Each contributed unique talents.

Kathleen Quinn entered this project at a critical point and had to restart the project from scratch. She helped me enormously during a difficult period when I was recovering from an accident and also trying to write critical chapters. Her experience and talents as a seasoned journalist proved invaluable in writing the commandments, 'Think Historically, Not Just Calorically', 'Separate Mood from Food' and 'Structure Gives Control'. Lee Quarfoot, a distinguished editor and journalist, assisted me in the writing of the preface, the commandment on strategy, 'Box It In, Box It Out', and the commandment on deprivation. Lee has endlessly shared professional guidance with me throughout this project. She is the consummate professional. Jim Gerard, a highly experienced journalist who has taught journalism at the university level, did much of the research and writing for my seminal commandment, 'The Problem May Be in the Food, Not in You', as well as contributing his talents to the writing and editing of other parts of the book. Bob Montgomery, a seasoned professional who has taught writing at one of the nation's leading universities, lent his considerable acumen and talents to 'Treat Your Calories Like Money', and 'Slips Should Teach You, Not Defeat You'. Bob also edited and rewrote critical aspects of this book, for which I owe him a great deal of gratitude.

I would like to thank David Nayor, a gifted health journalist who made monumental contributions to this book and its readers. David did the painstaking research, interviewing and nearly all the writing for the diet section and for 'Losing Weight Is Half the Job, Keeping It Off Is the Other Half'.

The Thin Commandments Diet is a tribute to the writing skills of these distinguished colleagues. I thank each of them.

On a personal note, I want to recognize a singular group of health professionals whose contributions to the advancement of medicine and the lives of their patients I admire greatly: Dr Ben Lewis, Dr Arnold Liscio, Dr Jimmie Holland, Dr David Peretz, Dr Orli Etingin, Dr Louis Aronne, Dr Artemis Simopoulos, Dr Eli Lizza, Dr Daniel Carr, Dr Jesse Rosenthal, Dr Sheenah Hankin and Dr William Suozzi. I owe a particular debt of great gratitude to Dr Daniel Baker, my friend and one of the world's pre-eminent plastic and reconstructive surgeons, who has helped me and so many others recover fully from the traumas of surgery for life-threatening illness. These individuals represent 'the best of the best' of American medicine and health care.

My acknowledgements for this book could never fail to mention a group of people I hold in great esteem: my clients. They are a truly enlightened group of people who appreciate that, in the end, it is not just about dieting but self-mastery over self-regret. Among them stand many of the brightest and toughest intellects of American society, men and women who have made an outstanding contribution to our world through their exemplary personal lives, the families they have shaped, and their leadership in guiding pre-eminent universities, teaching hospitals, major corporations and cultural and financial institutions. Some are fortunate enough to be the rich and famous and winners of Academy Awards and the prestigious prizes of the worlds of science and sports. But most are people just like you and me, who care deeply about the quality of their lives and who adamantly refuse to lose to a piece of food. They have been my greatest teachers, toughest reviewers and most enthusiastic supporters for more than a quarter century.

Lastly, I have only one regret – that my late mother, Rose Pernice Gullo, is not here to see this book. Through her love and caring, she has shaped all that I have done and will do in my life. My gratitude and respect for this woman I was blessed to call 'mother' is eternal.

Stephen Pernice Gullo
New York City
A.M.D.G.

Introduction

Calories are only half of the weight loss equation.

Now, welcome to the other half...

It has been said that the good doctor learns from his patients. My real education in the field of weight sciences began almost 25 years ago when I stopped looking at textbooks and prevailing theories for answers and starting *listening* to the men and women who came to me for help. It was only then that I realized why the standard approach to weight control was failing most people.

Earlier, as a student and then as a researcher and professor of human behaviour and health sciences at the Columbia-Presbyterian Medical Center, I had learned that a thorough medical and personal history is critical to accurate diagnosis and identifying effective treatments. As I met with more and more clients, it became clear that the field of weight control was missing this guiding principle of health care. Indeed, *weight control may be the only area of health care where history – in this case, the patient's unique food history – is completely ignored.*

By looking *historically* – not just calorically – at my clients' dieting, weight loss and weight gain, I saw that there were obstacles that repeatedly led these men and women down the path to failure. For some, it was a particular food. For some, it was a certain type of food, such as sweets or nibble foods. For others, it was a behavioural pattern, such as skipping meals or eating when they were bored or upset. When my patients incorporated new eating patterns, they would lose weight. When they returned to their old ways, control would be lost – and, like clockwork, the weight would come back. *They were gaining back the same weight with the same foods on the same days of the week at the same times over and over again. This was the one area of their lives where they were not learning from past mistakes!*

These individual patterns comprise what I call your Eating Print – the living history of the specific foods, situations, places and responses that make up the mosaic of your unique eating behaviours. *Your Eating Print is your own unique signature in the world of food.* Just like our fingerprints, everyone's Eating Print has distinctive characteristics, and once you know your Eating Print, you can predict your behaviour in any food situation, with any food. You can anticipate – and then prepare with strategy. Indeed, as I tell my own clients, once you know who you are in the world of food, you can predict how you will behave.

Unfortunately, every day millions of overweight people are given one-size-fits-all diets that directly contradict the lessons of their food history and Eating Prints. For example, the prevailing wisdom is that there are no good or bad foods. The statement is right, but the reasoning is wrong – *there are no good or bad foods; there are only good or bad histories with a food.* And *ignoring your personal history with such foods is what sets you up for failure.* It's quite simple: those who violate their food history fail, and those who honour their food history succeed. In this book, I will help you to understand the power of knowing your Eating Print and how to use these lessons to dramatically increase your success. I will teach you the critical concept that has changed my clients' approach to dieting forever. *When it comes to evaluating a food and its value for your weight control, think historically, not just calorically!* You will learn why history comes before calories in determining a food's suitability for your success at weight control.

When you break with the philosophy of dieting that thinks of calories alone and start to think historically, you individualize the world of food to your own past habits and unique eating patterns. The question, 'What is my history with this food (or this type of food)?' is a powerful mechanism to evaluate any food and a way to discover whether it will work for your success or against it. This fundamental shift in your thinking will change your perspective on the world of food forever. It is a shift that all my winners at weight control have made. We cannot possibly address in this book every food you have or will encounter, but once you make this shift in your thinking, you will have what I call 'the North Star' to guide you.

Diets succeed because they give structure to out-of-control eating and impose limits on foods. But once the diet is over, the boundaries are lifted and the limits are removed, sending people with weight problems out into the world with nothing but general guidelines on the importance of a 'balanced diet' and standard advice on enjoying their favourite foods 'in moderation'. This advice ignores the obvious fact that those who can eat moderately would not need a diet in the first place. Indeed, it's counter to the lessons of human history that in matters of pleasure and passion human beings are not given to moderation, but to excess. Can we really be surprised that so many people gain weight back?

If I could make one contribution to the field of weight control, it would be to make the field pay attention to food history. How can you expect a person to magically control a food or behaviour that's been out of control for decades? It's not enough to recommend moderation. You have to study that person's history and give them the skills to control what their history has shown to be problem areas.

THE OTHER HALF OF THE EQUATION...

Since its inception, the multibillion dollar weight loss industry has been dominated by scores of experts who have counselled over-weight people on what to eat and what not to eat. A single common focus has linked virtually every diet programme ever developed: an emphasis on calories, balancing them, limiting them and trying to burn them off. But I have broken away from this prevailing approach and have developed an entirely new paradigm for weight control – a paradigm *that emphasizes history before calories and replaces willpower with strategy – strategies that transform struggle into success. For strategy is stronger than willpower. It is this that makes success not only possible, but easy.* And unlike many weight programmes, the techniques and skills of the food strategy approach are truly universal, whether you're doing it alone, working with a nutritionist or dietitian, or following a commercial diet programme – from high protein/low carbohy-drate regimes like the Atkins Diet, to structured plans like Weight Watchers. This is the first weight control book to prove that – *with the right strategies – anyone can successfully manage their weight and make the fundamental shift from dieter to food strategist.*

The deeper I delved into my clients' histories, the clearer it became that it would take far more than nutritional advice and behaviour modification to conquer their strong social, biological and psychological programming. The traditional approach to weight control can't possibly address all these variables. In fact, it addresses only one – food and its calories.

A generation ago, perhaps, this model met a crying need. Our grandparents didn't understand the complexities of calories, carbohydrates, cholesterol and fats. But today we know which foods are good for our bodies and which foods undermine our health. *The problem facing this generation is not calories alone, but control.* That is why so many diet programmes fail. They focus almost exclusively on calorie management, while ignoring the destructive food programming of a lifetime. However, the purpose of this book is not just to share with you the best eating plan for safe and rapid weight loss or the 10 most crucial skills for success in weight control. It's about what few, if any, weight programmes have ever dealt with: how to change your fundamental thoughts and feelings about the very foods that have created your weight problem, so you're not always struggling with feelings of deprivation. If you're reading these words, chances are that you have lost weight many times, but you have never once changed your thinking about food.

But you have not been failing. Dieting has been failing you, by neglecting to teach you the strategies that you need to succeed. Without these, every one of your attempts at weight loss has been and will continue to be an unending struggle with willpower.

The 10 Per Cent Solution

The strategies that I will teach you in this book are not my own. They have been taught to me by the most powerful of all teachers – the thousands of my clients who have succeeded at weight control. They will help you not only to lose weight but also to change your thinking, so that you'll feel that you – not a biscuit or the bread bin – are calling the shots.

In *The Thin Commandments* I have distilled decades of my work and the lessons of the winners at weight control into the 10 most critical strategies for success at weight loss and the unique diet that makes it possible…and enjoyable.

Because of my early training in developmental and motivational psychology, my instinct has always been to focus on an individual's strengths rather than weaknesses. Early in my career, as I contemplated my clients' dilemmas, my thoughts turned to the minority of people who *do* succeed at weight loss, not only for the duration of their diet but also for years afterward. While success is defined differently in different studies – many use a low standard of keeping off just 5 pounds (2.25 kg) for only one year, which in my opinion isn't enough to define a lifestyle – the research with stringent standards suggests that somewhere between 3 and 10 per cent of dieters who manage to lose a significant amount of weight (at least 4.5–45 kg/10–100 lb) keep it off for five years or more.

For this elusive group – the real winners of weight loss – thin endures. I wondered what it is that they do that keeps them from becoming part of the 90 per cent or more who lose weight only to gain it back? And how could I use these insights to help those caught in the pattern of yo-yo dieting? *What is the 10 per cent solution?*

The answers to these questions are the message of *The Thin Commandments.*

Advertising Empowers Dieting

From the very start of my graduate studies, I have been fascinated by the motivational techniques of the advertising world and their power to change behaviour. Every day, advertisers convince millions of people to part with their money and to feel privileged. They reverse centuries of practical financial programming handed down to us through history (i.e. a penny saved is a penny earned), and lure us into buying things – expensive cars, designer trainers – for which we often have little if any need.

These campaigns succeed because they plant a new internal language and belief system in people who otherwise might not even care about the product. By repeating certain key ideas and slogans again and again, they instill a message; creating a very real and enduring psychological need for the advertiser's products. Sound familiar? 'Just do it', and 'I'll bet you can't eat just one'. No matter what the product may be, advertisers create a need for it that is so strong that it overrides another need – the need for money.

Food advertisers teach the very same lesson – that the smell, feel and taste of their foods are so compelling we need to have them, regardless of their cost to our health, looks and self-esteem.

I realized this same technique could be harnessed to overcome decades of food programming and could be used to motivate dieters to succeed.

In the months and years that followed this revelation, I began adapting the tools of advertising to the world of weight control and created a technique called *cognitive switching* (which I fully explain on page 138) and an allied strategy called *mental rehearsal* (discussed on page 140) to help my clients prepare in advance for any food situation. By employing these powerful techniques, they could even desensitize themselves to the allure of tempting foods and eliminate the cravings and feelings of deprivation.

I studied how dieters talk to themselves about food and identified key phrases that form the core of their 'food speak' – talk that creates a powerful need to eat certain foods and stirs up cravings and feelings of deprivation if they're not consumed. I created and taught my clients a new script that replaced the old 'food speak' and showed them a new way to think about food. Through cognitive switching and mental rehearsal, simple techniques that you will soon master, my clients learned a new language and new way to become winners at weight control! They were empowered to put their need to be trim and look good before their need for food – even the foods that had sabotaged all their previous weight control efforts.

The Best Diet

Historically, one of the most frequently heard complaints is that diet programme foods don't taste good. In 2005, that is a complete myth, especially in view of the world of food we now inhabit. In the decade since I wrote my first book, *Thin Tastes Better* the whole universe of food has changed. We're now living in a veritable paradise that includes a miracle cracker that kills appetite yet contains only 18 calories: fat-free natural yogurt that tastes great; and luscious chocolate mousses that contain a surprisingly small amount of calories. Supermarkets, health food stores and gourmet food shops now stock diet products that can give you all the taste you want...without the calories. When you use these foods, you can enjoy your fill and never feel deprived...for dieting is no longer about deprivation but substitution.

Time and time again, clients have told me that their success would have been impossible without these diet foods, which made success at weight control a pleasure instead of a struggle. Most significant, through the quick and easy recipes, you'll enjoy 5-star dining without the calories.

It is the only diet programme in the world designed not only on the basis of calories, carbs and grams of fat but also around *your* behaviour and food preferences. It teaches you not only which are the best foods for weight loss but also how to predict which foods are most likely to sabotage your success. Now you can select foods on the basis of calories and your ability to succeed on this diet. And through the vehicle of the unique 'new scale', *you will have the only tool in the world of weight control that can predict which of your day-to-day behaviours are early warning signs of problems ahead and how to quickly avoid them.*

The strategies I'm about to share with you have been featured in over 20 national and international cover stories in the US, including a *New York Times* Lifestyle section article that recognized my success rate as far surpassing any known standards in the diet industry. Through the pages of this book, you will learn the unique strategies and the central part of the eating plan, for which my clients have waited up to a year for an appointment. Perhaps this is one of the greatest testimonies to the power and effectiveness of what you will read herein.

Unlike diet books that just tell you about what works to lose weight, I will also tell you about what works for the psyche, what makes it easy to stay with this diet, and what works for real people who live life on the go. *The Thin Commandments is the missing link in the gap between knowing what to do and knowing how to do it.* For those who struggled with their weight, it's the key that can unlock the door to permanent weight loss.

In this book, I will take you through these simple strategies step-by-step, guiding you along the path that has brought so many people to their personal, permanent thin. Through the use of these creative and winner-tested strategies, you will learn to do things in a new way – an easier way – and get a new result: success.

No matter how many times you failed in the past, and regardless of all the setbacks, remember that you have never given up. You have always held on to that desire for success. And how strong and powerful that desire must be! You and I together 'will find a way, or make one'. I have seen it work for thousands of people; *for dieting is about losing weight…food strategy is about ending the problem!*

BEYOND DIETING: YOUR LIFE FACTOR

I want you to think about why you bought this book. It wasn't just to read words on a page, learn my philosophy of weight control or even fit into your clothes. On the most fundamental level, you bought this book because there was a discomfort or unhappiness in your life. An unhappiness with your weight, your appearance, the fit of your clothes, the amount of control food exercised over you, and the way you were dealing with it. Through these pages, you will find the path to remove this unhappiness and in its place improve your appearance and enhance your health and the quality of your life. This is the blessing that you will give to yourself.

To eat according to the principles of this book is not about dieting; it's about being food-smart and life-smart. It takes dieting out of the old association with deprivation and puts it into the larger context of your life. It is about the quality of your life – looking younger and living longer, at the top of your game.

This book is, in the end, about empowerment, and that most elusive of all human goals – happiness.

I joke with my clients that when I'm 80 and in God's waiting room, when everyone else is taking the Prozac of the day, I'll be making the rounds of all the pizzerias and bakeries. In fact, I plan to leave this world in a pizza truck!

In the meantime, none of us wants to look back to the prime of our lives when we had our youthfulness, attractiveness and health and realize that we squandered it all to hang out with a biscuit tin, a bag of sweets or a pizza. This is the greatest deprivation of all.

There's a powerful line in Elton John and Tim Rice's Broadway hit, *Aida*: 'We are given paradise, but only for a day.' And though our lives aren't paradise, we have the power and the privilege to make them better and to appreciate what is truly meaningful and eternal. This is our 'day'.

In the end, you must face the truth: you have seen and tasted it all in the world of food. It has not made you happy; it has only made you heavy. There has got to be a better way. This book is the better way.

PART I

THE THIN COMMANDMENTS

Dieting is about losing weight — food strategy is about ending the problem.

The First Thin Commandment:
Strategy Is Stronger Than Willpower

COMMANDMENT ESSENTIALS

- Use strategy to stay in control.
- Stop self-defeating food talk.
- Weigh yourself on the New Scale for Dieting.
- Keep a food diary.
- Listen to a power tape.

THE SINGLE GREATEST SURPRISE of my professional life has been the discovery that success at weight control is *not* about willpower. Indeed, those who succeed at weight control do not have greater willpower than those who fail — they just have better strategies. This is the most powerful lesson I have learned in 25 years from almost 15,000 clients.

Like you — and many of my colleagues — I once had quite a few preconceptions about people with weight problems: they lack willpower to control their eating; they have psychological or emotional issues that keep them from permanently losing weight; and they lack the knowledge to follow a healthy diet.

When I actually began to work with these individuals, I

discovered that almost all of my preconceptions were wrong. They were successful in their professional lives, enjoyed many interests and had meaningful personal relationships. They were creative people with vision, who cared passionately about their goals and were dedicated to excellence. They epitomized the American ideal of determination and success.

Far from lacking nutritional knowledge, many of my clients already knew *what* to eat and what *not* to eat. They'd read diet book after diet book, were aware of calories, carbohydrates and fats, and knew how to read labels. Many had lost hundreds of pounds over the years. But despite all their knowledge and weight loss, they had never been able to keep the pounds off permanently.

I struggled to reconcile my clients' success in every other area of their lives with their failure at weight control. How could these people – many of whom had overcome tremendous obstacles to achieve greatness – still lose control with chocolates or a bread-basket? They knew what they had to do to lose weight, but they were living in misery because they couldn't do it. Such repeated failure takes a terrible toll, even on the most successful individual.

WHY WE FAIL

By looking back across the years at my clients' dieting, weight loss and gain, I've seen that *there are distinct and predictable patterns of behaviour and food choices that have led these men and women to failure.* I have conclusively discovered that the particular diet an individual follows is secondary to success at weight control, which is why people can so easily switch diets from year to year. The most important factor for winning is having strategies – not the particular diet you follow.

In a recent article 'The Diet That Works' in the *Wall Street Journal*, Tara Parker Pope captured the truth that resonates for a large number of individuals who struggle with weight control. 'If sticking to a diet were easy, so many of us wouldn't be so fat.'

The men and women who *have* avoided a weight problem – or conquered one on their own – instinctively use strategy to stay in control. It's the common thread that unites everyone who has ever won at weight control, including myself. Food strategy has saved me again and again in my own life.

Obviously, no one who has lost weight intends to gain it back. After every diet, every one of my clients was completely committed to maintaining his or her weight loss. But the commitment was overcome by a combination of powerful forces: biology, our value system and advertising.

Recent research shows that our ancestors passed on powerful biological programming that may predispose us to crave and seek out certain foods, as many of us who are sensitive to sweet, salty and bitter tastes know well. *These differences in sensitivity, not willpower, may explain why some people are able to maintain control around certain foods – such as chocolate chip cookies – while others find that these foods actually trigger increased appetite and losses of control.*

And unlike many of our ancestors, who had to struggle to find food, we are literally surrounded by it. Yet we still carry the ancestral mindset of 'waste not, want not' in our modern society where food is overly abundant and always present. Just consider all of the supermarkets, fast-food chains, shopping centre takeaways and convenience stores. Food is everywhere and we can virtually eat whatever we want, whenever we want. We're also bombarded by slick commercials that reinforce the belief that foods are the goodies and treats that make life worthwhile and wash away stress – and that any limitation of them is a horrible deprivation. Even the language of love is expressed in terms of food – honey, cookie, peaches, sweetie.

Saddled with this powerful psychological and biological programming, surrounded by messages that food is the answer to every problem and the reward for every success, it's no wonder so many people fall back into the habits that lead to weight gain. And it's totally clear why so many feel instantly deprived when they think about weight control.

STRATEGY: THE KEY PRINCIPLES

Food situations are a part of every life. They come up again and again, and there's an amazing amount of predictability to what you can expect to encounter. Most of us rely on a very small assortment of foods – the same vegetables, the same meats, the same snack foods that satisfy an eat-and-run diet. Despite the fact that we can buy practically any food at any time, no matter how exotic or out of season, few of us venture beyond the limits of our favourite foods. And most eating occurs in only about seven situations: at home, in the workplace, in restaurants, in others' homes, when travelling, on holiday, and at celebratory events, such as weddings and parties. *The realm of food is not a big world, but a small village.*

The same scenarios come up over and over again. You face the same foods, the same temptations. However overwhelmed you may feel in the land of abundance, there is another more powerful truth at work as well: you have seen it all and tasted it all before. It may come in different shapes, varieties and new presentations, but there's very little that's new in the world of food that you will face today. I will teach you strategies to deal with each situation. And I'll show you ways to develop your skills so that your responses become automatic. Rather than a constant tug-of-war that drains your willpower and resolve, you will have a set of tools to rely on, no matter where you go or what foods you may meet along the way.

Although food strategies vary depending on the person, the techniques share common themes. This chapter and those that follow will teach you a new way of dealing with your weight that involves key principles that have enabled so many of my clients to turn a lifetime of failure with weight into a lifetime of success.

• **Food history.** In a world of thousands of types of food, my careful research has revealed that only a handful are at the root of most weight problems. Food history shows that weight control is not a mountain to climb, just a few patterns to master.

• **Food desensitizing.** Techniques to defuse the power of cravings so that you can be around food that would normally tempt you without feeling deprived.

• **Breaking through food 'baby talk'.** Methods to transform self-defeating food talk learned in childhood – that can rule and ruin adulthood – into a new script, with phrases, thoughts and values that work in the real world and prove that anyone can overcome feelings of deprivation.

• **The New Scale for Dieting.** A unique and effective tool for measuring the shifts and changes in your attitudes, skills and motivation that can result in increased pounds, to be used as an early warning system *before* you step on a real scale. *The New Scale for Dieting predicts in advance if you'll be gaining weight* and makes it possible to prevent the seven most critical mistakes that lead to weight gain. This has never before been done in a weight programme.

• **Containment.** The powerful technique that turns slips into success and teaches you how to cut off an error and never again feel the guilt of 'I blew it'.

• **Keeping the pleasure of food.** Enjoying favourite foods and not feeling deprived is critical to your success. Through recipes and food preparation techniques in my diet plan, you'll discover how to preserve the joy of eating without excess calories. And the gourmet recipes will prove that success at weight control is not about giving up the pleasure of fine dining. Indeed, *not* to enjoy the foods on a weight plan guarantees failure!

Whenever I teach new clients the techniques for weight control, I know that I am training them for 'diet fitness'. For, just as you can become physically fit and train for a sport, every overweight person has the ability to become psychologically fit and train for long-term weight control. These strategies, along with many others that I will teach you, make it possible not only to dramatically increase your likelihood of success on a diet but also to maintain that success for years.

Some of these strategies may seem unusual or contradict what you have been led to believe about dieting and weight control. But successful weight control is not about doing what's 'normal' – it's about doing what works for you. You should not be concerned about the norm – that's the preoccupation of the insecure – but about what brings you the success you deserve. As Chairman Deng responded when criticized by the Communist hardliners for introducing capitalist initiatives into China, 'It doesn't matter if the cat is black or white; it only matters if it can catch mice.'

DIETS ARE JUST WORDS ON A PAGE

Most of the diet books out there today focus on only half the equation: the right foods. *But that leaves out the most critical element of success – you!* Diets are just words on a page, a list on paper of what to eat. They don't help you plan what to think or say, and they certainly don't tell you how to *behave*. They ignore the right behaviours, the critical issues of how to stay motivated and how to bounce back from a lapse, and how to avoid cravings and feelings of deprivation, and they don't change your thinking about food.

Strategy deals with how to make weight control easy. The right techniques actually encourage you to *want* to continue. They lead you to a way of eating that makes you feel happier and brings about permanent results by changing your mindset. At the core of the lessons I teach is changing the food programming that you've been taught since childhood.

The Lure of Food 'Baby Talk'

When faced with cravings and feelings of deprivation, most dieters slide straight back into childhood – and that language that goes with it. 'But it's my favourite.' 'It's not fair that I can't have it.' 'But I've been so good.' 'It's my comfort.' 'It's my treat.' 'I'll reward myself.' This food 'baby talk' is at the heart of many people's weight problems, drowning out their common sense and even their desire for health and sometimes life itself.

For many of my clients, this is the only area in their lives still run by the childhood patterns of thinking and conditioning. Indeed, for so many of us, it is the single area of living where childhood thinking has never been updated. *Where food is concerned, even the most mature adults often act like children – like children who want their way no matter what, blocking out the negative consequences of their eating.* They focus instead on a few minutes' worth of taste that fills the mouth and lingers for a short while, while completely denying the obvious and discomforting cost.

For these foods are not free – you have to wear them for years to come. You can't eat it all and still be thin. This is a fact. But you can be a selective gourmet and never have to give up the pleasure of fine dining. Food is everywhere, and because it so often looks and tastes great, it's easy for us to continue to live in this childish mindset, telling ourselves 'these are my goodies and treats'. And we often listen to the message – until it creates disaster. The challenge is that the food is immediate, but the cost is often paid in the long term.

And like most long-term payment plans, the interest is high. Perhaps you have only to look in the mirror?

Only children live their lives believing they can have it all without any cost. Now it's time for you to bring this part of your life into the adult world. All of life contains adjustments and trade-offs. In accepting this, you not only establish a framework for lasting solutions to your weight problem, but you become a more resilient and mature human being. *It's time to stop resenting what you do to keep your body healthy and attractive.* Everything you value in your life – your relationships, your children and your career – has taken work, focus and endurance. Why should it be any different when it comes to managing your weight? Strategy, however, minimizes the cost and maximizes the reward.

The winners have come to this realization, and they no longer feel deprived, but liberated. In a recent survey of my clients, 86 per cent said they felt no sense of deprivation. Without taking this step of growth and maturation, there can be no permanent weight loss, no permanent freedom. They've taken a turn in their evolution – evolving from childhood thinking and values into the adult thinking in the world of foods.

If you've come this far, you are already well on your way to that understanding and sense of freedom. You bought this book because you want to lose weight, and you want to do better at ongoing weight control. Now the choice to act is yours.

THREE SIMPLE STEPS

There are three actions that can encourage your progress, guard it and enhance it. For thousands of my clients, these have proven to be among the most effective weapons available for arming themselves in their battle with weight. They reinforce all of the messages of this book, and I encourage you to do all three of them.

Weigh Yourself on the New Scale for Dieting

Scales don't keep people thin. Every heavy person owns a set of scales. It is the measure that tells us just how far we've strayed from thin. The weight scale is the end result of your behaviours; it reports where you have stood with the foods in your life since you last weighed in. The New Scale for Dieting predicts in advance which direction the weight scale will be moving – it provides an early warning system. The New Scale for Dieting is a simple 10-question quiz (see the opposite page) that reviews the basic skills and attitudes that you should be maintaining as part of your healthy life of thin. With it, you can track changes in your control skills and thinking in the same way that a diabetic tracks blood sugar or someone with hypertension monitors blood pressure. With regular use, it can alert you to areas where you may be weak and therefore vulnerable to slip-ups and bring your behaviour and thinking in line with the winners at weight control. *The questions reflect the actions of those who succeed at weight control. In weighing yourself on the New Scale for Dieting, you have an instant means of knowing that you are on the same path.* I tell my clients to weigh themselves once a week on a weight scale and once a week on the New Scale for Dieting. This is to guide you to your goal. Once you reach your maintenance level, and the weight scale is no longer going down every week, your motivation will change, and you'll need another, modified New Scale (you'll find it on page 184) to use for quizzing yourself regularly, to protect all that you've accomplished.

Keep a Food Diary

In the studies on weight control, one factor keeps recurring: *those who maintain a written record of what they're eating each day lose more weight and do significantly better at keeping it off than those who do not.* A food diary that tracks what and when you eat will allow you to detect any problems in your eating plan as they occur and to accurately gauge how much you are consuming. There is nothing else you can do that takes just a few minutes a day that will increase your weight loss and the likelihood of success as much as this.

I recommend keeping your food diary in a notebook beside your bed, where you can record in it, morning and night. Write down everything you eat, and I mean *everything*, including any nibbles. To help identify your patterns, circle your errors: foods that you may have eaten in excessive amounts, foods not on your eating plan and foods with hidden calories, such as those cooked in oil, butter or sauces.

You might also find that it gives you an extra edge to plan meals in advance. You'll benefit from writing out the next day's menus and snacks – especially if it's a day when you expect to be stressed out or to face an array of food temptations, or if you've seen some recent slippage and need to get back on the right footing and follow

The New Scale for Dieting

Do this quiz about once a week. If you're falling back into old patterns and an old foodie belief system, this exercise will make you aware of it. The commandments in this book are designed to help you get it right. Every time you ask these questions, your psyche gets the message about the behaviours and thinking that are becoming a natural part of your new lifestyle.

1. Am I going more than 3 to 4 hours without a healthy snack or meal?

2. Am I failing to plan (i.e., letting supplies of healthy foods run out, going into food situations hungry, failing to prepare for high-risk food situations, and failing to carry my ThinPack when travelling or going out for a busy day)? (See Chapter 4 for more on ThinPacks.)

3. Am I avoiding foods I have a long history of abusing?

4. Am I keeping my moods out of my foods? Am I not eating out of boredom or anger, and am I reminding myself in stressful situations that 'this is not about food'?

5. Am I keeping problem foods out of the house or out of sight?

6. Am I avoiding high-risk situations (i.e., reading dessert menus, dining in restaurants with buffet-style service)?

7. Am I maintaining finger control? Avoiding mindless nibbling?

8. Am I eating too much of the 'right foods' (such as chicken or fruit) on my plan?

9. Am I watching for the hidden calories that stop weight loss (such as those found in salad dressings, foods made in butter or oil, sauces on food, and side dishes), and failing to ask in restaurants 'what does it come with?' and 'how's it prepared?'

10. Am I reminding myself that this is not about deprivation but doing what works for a happier, healthier life?

through. The advance notice programmes the psyche and structures behaviour. It works like an early fire-alarm system.

Listen to a Power Tape

Would you like to get the same training that my clients receive without paying thousands of dollars? Would you like to get the same benefits?

Making a recording, in any way that suits your lifestyle – on a cassette, CD or any other electronic means – and listening to it frequently utilizes one of the most powerful techniques that I have adapted from the advertising world – that is, to reinforce a message by repeating certain key ideas and phrases again and again. It's a powerful tool not only for your behaviour but for changing your lifelong thinking and feeling about food. As an instrument for weight control, it will push your buttons to motivate the behaviour you want and extinguish the behaviour you don't want. As you read this book, pick out several of the commandments – or go for all of them – to use in making tapes for yourself.

A food-control cassette is one of the surefire ways to quell cravings, short-circuit a sense of deprivation and reinforce motivation and commitment. Basically, your tapes are an advertising campaign for you, and the product they are pitching is a new you. And like any successful ad campaign, they need to be upbeat, catchy and full of powerful images that will capture your imagination and interest. In this chapter and the ones that follow, I've given you tips for writing your own scripts and three sample dialogues to help you through the three most critical moments in weight control:

1. Getting started

2. Keeping your motivation high, especially once you pass the midpoint of your weight loss, and you're starting to look and feel better

3. Adjusting to the lifestyle for maintenance

As you listen to the tapes regularly, your mind will absorb the message and start reinforcing it on its own, and your thought patterns will begin to mimic the ideas on the tapes. After just a few weeks of daily listening, you should begin to hear the words of your new food talk spontaneously. The repetition will begin to become your internal self-talk, and the changes will be seen not only in your attitude but also in your behaviour with food.

Your cassette or CD is a cheerleader in your pocket, always there to give support. You can listen to it in your car on your way to work, or in the bathroom while you shave or shower in the morning, or while power walking. You can draw on the tape at any time to help drown out the old food talk and reinforce your new inner dialogue.

Your recordings should be as unique and individual as you are. The scripts should be tailored to suit your own situation. You may find it more powerful to speak in the first person, saying, 'I will start living today as I never have before!' Or, if a coaching tone works better for you, you might consider using the second-person: '*You* will start your food-control programme today!' Write your scripts to accommodate your needs.

Once you have your library of food talk tapes, make sure you listen to them every day. While you're losing weight and even after you've reached your goal, don't stop tuning in. You don't have to listen every day, but don't cut them out completely. The biggest threat to your weight control is to get cocky and think you're cured. Thin is a lifestyle – not some arbitrary number on a scale. Remember, *you lose the weight; you don't lose the vulnerability.*

Play It Again...and Again...and Again

A food diary and a food-control recording are among the strongest weapons you have in your weight-loss arsenal, a frontline defence in the battle for control over your body. Don't underestimate their power. Writing a message *and* hearing a message over and over again sinks that message indelibly into your conscious and subconscious mind. The tapes are designed to drown out the old messages that food is sending you – 'I have to have it. It looks so delicious. It's so interesting' – and to empower you and keep you focused in challenging situations, such as when you're under stress or bored. The diary and tapes can keep you from falling into the pattern of doing what you've always done.

Repetition is one of the most powerful tools of advertising.

(continued on page 38)

Sample Tape No. 1: Getting Started

Make listening to a tape a part of your routine. Hearing the messages in the morning can be especially effective, getting you off on the right foot to face the day and follow through. This script will help to get you started. Edit it however it suits you to address your vulnerabilities and reprogramme your thinking.

You may feel a bit awkward at first as you speak into the tape recorder. But like so many aspects of food control, the consistent and faithful repetition of the process makes it easier and easier to do.

- 'What is wrong with this picture of my life that I am losing to a piece of food, taking orders from a bar of chocolate (or whatever your problem foods may be)?'
- 'I will start my food plan today. I don't want to wait. I won't say that I'll start eating well tomorrow. How many times have I said that before? Saying tomorrow is saying I will *not* do it today. *This* is the tomorrow I spoke of yesterday. I would never run a business the way I've treated my own body and my weight problem. If this were something that I needed to do for my children or someone I love, I would have done it a long time ago. Now, indeed, I will do

it for someone I love – myself.'
- 'Today, I'll start living as never before. I'll remember that thin begins in the supermarket. I will buy the foods that support my success and avoid the ones that sabotage it. If I don't buy it, I don't eat it. If it's not in my kitchen, it's not on my hips.'
- Remind yourself why you're doing this. 'None of my clothes fit. I can't bear to look at a picture of myself or in the mirror. I'm not taking care of my health or the quality of my life.'
- Talk about the journey. 'There's not a single food that I'll see today that I haven't seen or tasted before. I have seen it all, I've tasted it all, and it hasn't made me happy; it has only made me heavy. This is not a mountain to climb. It is just a few patterns to master. I have overcome a great deal in my life. I can learn to manage three meals and two or three snacks a day. That is my only challenge – to buy a lifetime of being trim. What's the worst that can happen to me? I will just see or smell a food that I'd like to eat. It will not be new. I have seen and tasted it before. A food temptation is simply a feeling, it's not a

command. It lasts about 4 to 12 minutes. If I break the eye contact and say "No way!" it will pass. Isn't thin worth 4 to 12 minutes of standing up to a feeling?'

- Remind yourself of your history. 'What I have done in the past has not worked. That's why I will do it a new way using strategy. If it seemed difficult in the past, it probably was because I didn't have strategy. I knew what I wanted – to be trim – but I didn't have a plan to get there and stay there. Strategy gives me the road map that makes it possible. It's not just knowing what to eat and what not to eat. It's knowing how to do it, how to want to do it and how to make it easy to do. That's what strategy is about, and that's what I'm working on, one day at a time.'

- Focus on the foods and the habits that have contributed to your weight problem. Name your problem foods and behaviours. If you've decided that certain foods have made you fail repeatedly, and you want to avoid them while you're trying to lose weight, be very clear and strong with yourself. Either say you are going to temporarily avoid these foods, or you are going to limit them to spe-

cial situations. If you've decided to limit specific foods by reserving them for certain times or places, say to yourself, 'I will only eat them on Sunday night…or never in a restaurant and never at home.'

- If you are a stress eater, be sure to remind yourself that food doesn't solve problems. 'If I have an upsetting situation, I will say to myself, I have an uncomfortable feeling, but it is not about food. Eating over it will not make me happy; it will only make me heavy. Even if I can't solve the problem or change the person who is upsetting me, by not eating, I break a major pattern that has made me heavy. Maybe I can't do anything about other problems in my life, but my weight is one area that I have the power to change. And I will use that power.'

- End with empowerment and perspective. 'In a world where there is cancer, and AIDS, and homelessness, what's the big deal if I say no thanks to (problem food), so I can say yes to being thin? Did I come this far in life to take orders from a (problem food)?' Remind yourself of your power. 'I deserve to be trim. I deserve to succeed with this. I deserve to be in control in my life with food.'

Throughout this book, I'll be repeating key phrases over and over again. This is by intent, to help you change your thinking, not just to have you read words and forget them. Together, we'll use techniques to enhance your life and sell you on a new, thin, all-you-can-be you!

DISCOVER WHERE YOU STAND

Weight loss, like most things in life, occurs in stages, over time. Different thoughts, emotions and levels of motivation mark each stage. For most dieters, feelings of ambivalence and indecisiveness toward old food temptations start to surface after a while. You may diet for many weeks without a hint of a doubt, untroubled by any seductive signals from favourite foods or old eating habits. But then you can begin to waver.

More than likely, you've reached one of the critical, problematic spots of dieting. To maintain your weight – and your control over food – you need to be aware of where you stand in this progression of stages. When you truly know who you are, where you are and how you perform in the world of food, you can predict how you will behave – and, if necessary, take steps to remain on track and to bolster your flagging motivation and confidence.

Sometimes, after an initial rapid weight loss, the weight drop starts to slow, and you can become discouraged. That's the time to recall that your new programme isn't just about losing pounds or kilos, it's about losing the problem of yo-yo dieting. Another danger is that, sometimes, after the weight starts to come off, and the clothes get loose, you may develop the misconception that you are already thin, when, in fact, you are simply a little less overweight. The truth is, it's easy to delude yourself, to think because your weight is less, your vulnerability is less and your need for the strategies is less. On the contrary, strategy becomes more important as a dieter progresses through the phases, and it is most critical in the final phase of maintenance.

Losing weight doesn't change your history, your taste buds or your vulnerability, so it's essential to avoid becoming sloppy with the strategies or the planning – that's the first critical lesson to master: *think strategy.*

The Three Most Critical Points in a Diet Plan

In working with my clients, I've found three stages in the process of weight control that pose the greatest risk of derailing a weight programme and undermining a new eating lifestyle. Navigating through these challenges is the path to truly mastering your control with food.

• **At the beginning.** The motivation to start dieting often begins with a desire to look better, to fit into your clothes, to feel better about yourself and to improve your health – and it often means experiencing strong, very negative feelings. You may feel disgusted with yourself for your lack of control, or hate to look at yourself in the mirror, or dread opening your wardrobe because you have nothing to wear that will make you feel good about yourself. Although this is the stage that propels many overweight people into treatment, it can also become a black hole, in which motivation to change is overwhelmed by a sense of futility and self-loathing. This is why it's so important to get started with a belief in yourself and your own ability to succeed. I frequently remind my clients that it's just a piece of food against them. Food has no intelligence or strategy. It has no I.Q. You have every advantage when you know yourself, your history and how to approach food situations.

• **At the midpoint.** There's a natural tendency to become less careful when you've started to succeed. Most people on a weight programme start to see significant changes in 10 to 30 days. You don't even need to get to the end, to your ideal weight, to see the reward. Your clothes are looser, you're getting compliments, you're happier with yourself, your pain has gone away, and suddenly, you're sliding into old patterns, sabotaging yourself. You may believe that because you've lost a bit of weight, you've lost your control problems with certain foods. You may forget that just because the weight starts to come off, it doesn't mean your history, your taste buds or your vulnerability to your trigger or problematic foods has changed. Perhaps you're telling yourself that you can handle 'just a little'. You're feeling a lot less urgency to watch yourself with quantities, to plan ahead, to shop carefully. You become complacent – and complacency is the enemy of thin. Fortunately, there are strategies to save you.

● **At the end.** Success is yours! You've reached your personal best. Every time you look in the mirror, you feel a thrill of pleasure and a sense of pride. The intense satisfaction of achieving your treasured goal convinces you that you'll never go back to your old ways again. Your motivation and commitment are high – for a while. But soon, the honeymoon is over, and you've got to get down to the business of living trim. Maintenance is the most high-risk period of any weight-control effort. Lots of people succeed with dieting – they get an A for dieting every time they stay the course – and then they flunk maintenance. The cause, of course, is usually a lapse in the strategies that are designed not only to carry you through but to help you realize that just because you've lost the weight, you haven't lost the problem.

Many people think about achieving their weight goal in the same way they think about achieving good high school grades – you get them once and then you can take them for granted for the rest of your life. But food control is an ongoing, dynamic process. And to make the transition from dieting to lifestyle mode requires changing your thinking and staying with the strategies, which will give you the tools for life, to maintain a lifetime of trim.

A Periodic Checkup

For the record, thin doesn't mean qualifying for the cover of *GQ, Shape* or *Fitness* magazines. By thin, I simply mean your 'personal thin'. For some, that's the ideal number on the medical charts. For others, personal thin may not be that number – though my wish for each of you is that your weight should be in a healthy range. Yet I realize that if a person is 22 kg (50 lb) overweight, and he is motivated or able to lose only 4–10 kg (10–20 lb), right now, his life will still be healthier – and this is his personal thin for now.

Throughout this book, when I use the word *fat*, I do not mean it as a judgement, nor as a derogatory term. Fat is simply the word that refers to being medically obese, and I do not attach any judgement to it.

THE WORK OF HAPPINESS

You probably have always associated diets with deprivation. There is a way around this stumbling block. Put it in the larger context of your life and your most treasured goal − to be happy. It may seem strange in the First Commandment of this book, when there is so much to say about weight control, that I want to talk about the work of happiness. What, you may ask, does that have to do with your losing some weight and getting back into your clothes? But from my point of view, happiness and weight loss are very important and intimately connected. The popular mantra of the diet industry is all foods in moderation, but that's a tough trick to pull off when the world we live in isn't given to moderation. It's not enough to want to be trim. You need a plan to get there and stay there. A plan that's livable and doable and that you'll enjoy following − a plan that is about the work of happiness − the happiness that comes from living the vision you have for your own body.

Foods may give you momentary pleasure, but your happiness is the greater reward when you look in the mirror and know you're looking your best, wearing clothes that you've always wanted to wear, feeling fit and glowing with well-being. In our fast-paced culture, the landscape of food is always evolving. In recent decades, the level of food stimuli has increased dramatically. To live in this world and be what I call a selective gourmet − not a compulsive eater − involves strategy.

The role of strategy is to save the foods you love the most and keep them in your life. And it also can let you keep what you care about the most − your appearance, your clothes, your control and your good health.

As you read the pages of this book and approach your weight-control efforts, stop thinking about dieting. This is what I tell my clients when they first enter my office. It surprises them, until I go on to say that they should *think instead about looking 10 years younger without a face-lift, think in terms of quality of life, self-mastery and growth, fashionable clothes, saving guilt hours at the gym, struggling to make up for yesterday's food excesses. Most of all, I tell them, think about life enhancement − extending and enjoying every day to come of the lives they've been given. I tell them they should think about their highest goals and the work of happiness.*

There is a simple and powerful truth that I will repeat again and again throughout this book: *being thin may not make you happy, but being fat will make you unhappy.* I can say that on the darkest day of your life, you'll always be happier with yourself if you are living in control with your weight and your food. And I can also say that if you look at the broader picture, *not* living trim and in control will always be harder. Always failing with your weight, never knowing success, always feeling reluctant to face yourself in the mirror or a camera – this is far harder than saying no to the breadbasket, a piece of cake, or any food.

The goal of the strategies that I present here is not just to change your weight, or change your size, or even to change your behaviour – but to change, on the most fundamental level, your thinking. So it's easy to follow all of the other commandments!

There are no good or bad foods.
There are only good or bad histories with a food.

The Second Thin Commandment:
Think Historically,
Not Just Calorically

COMMANDMENT ESSENTIALS

- Think about your food history – how you've behaved with 'problem foods' in the past.
- Identify trigger foods, behaviours, situations and times that lead you to lose control of your eating.
- Stop thinking about simply counting calories, but about how much of your problem food you eat at any one time.
- Realize that even most 'healthy' foods aren't healthy if you eat too much of them.

STARTING RIGHT NOW, this book will do something no other diet book has done for you before: it will change your *thinking* about what you eat, and it will change it for the rest of your life.

THE MISSING LINK

Ever since the word 'dieting' has been in our language, it has been synonymous with calories and calorie counting. We are taught to think *calorically* about losing weight, and more recently, people are being taught to count the grams of carbohydrates as well. Yet it is this very emphasis on thinking about calories and now carbohydrates that has led millions and millions of people who are successful in so many other things in life to fail utterly at dieting!

Thinking calorically is focusing on the food: what's in the food and how it behaves in your body. Thinking *historically* is all about you: how *you* have behaved with this food over the years of your life and the unique history you have with any food. The problem with the traditional dieting approach is that it is entirely focused on the food: how many calories, how many grams of carbohydrates, how many grams of fat and so on. Thinking historically shifts the focus to the most critical element for diet success − *you*.

This is the missing link for weight control.

Two people may have a very different history or response to a single 100-calorie cookie. For one person, the cookie may be satisfying − so much so that the person has never abused cookies in his life. For someone else, that one cookie may trigger them to want more and more and even binge on the whole packet. Knowing which is true for you may ultimately prove more important to your long-term success at weight control than knowing that the cookie has 100 calories.

When you think historically, you use your whole life experience to evaluate food. Your whole life experience is an immediate predictor of how you will next behave with this food. No weight-control programme could possibly discuss every single food you will encounter on your road through life. But by using your own history with food, you have an almost perfect guide.

All you need to do is shift your thinking and ask yourself, 'What is my history with this food or this type of food?'

YOUR PERSONAL HISTORY WITH FOOD

Stop and think for a moment what happens whenever you register with a new doctor: he will request the records from your previous doctor. Before any doctor attempts a diagnosis, and especially before he prescribes any treatment for you, that doctor wants to know your unique medical history, along with a description of the nature and severity of your symptoms. Only then can you be put on the right path to recovery and lasting health.

As I said in the introduction, *weight control may be the only area of health care where a person's unique food history is totally ignored.* And the consequences have been disastrous. As a professional, it's extremely painful to realize that the dieting field, in its very attempt to help people, has actually led millions and millions – and probably you, the reader – to failure. The need to understand an individual's history with food is the most obvious need in the field of weight control but, tragically, it is the one most overlooked.

The book you have in your hands is the only weight programme in the world that teaches you that knowing your own eating history is *first* when it comes to weight control. It comes before learning any calorie tables. For the first time, your eating history is given equal footing with the calories in foods – and this book will explain that in certain situations, respecting your food history is far more important than avoiding excess calories in deciding what to eat.

Every day, weight-control programmes and bestselling diet books prescribe one-size-fits-all diets that blatantly violate dieters' food histories. These programmes set up dieters for failure, even though they all have only the best intentions. The fact that the vast majority of all people who diet regain the weight they lost is powerful evidence that there is something terribly wrong with the standard approach and recommendations that diet planners and diet books make. If I could make one contribution to the field of weight control, it would be to make the entire field *pay attention to food history* as a central guiding principle.

This is not intended as criticism of my colleagues, who have contributed enormously in the effort to help end obesity. We are all victims of our training, and those who are trained alike, think alike. Fortunately, for the first time in the history of weight control, there really is a dramatic new principle to guide the field: *think historically, not just calorically.* We can now combine what we know about nutrition, calories, the human body and human behaviour to think in a new way about weight control.

THE KEY TO SUCCESS

When I first started out in the field of weight control, I, like everyone else, thought calorically instead of historically in approaching weight loss. But I was extremely lucky that I soon acquired for a client a very insightful woman named Joan, who runs a very important charity in New York City. Despite all her intelligence, her virtues and her skills, Joan actually thought of herself as weak-willed and even occasionally 'bad' because no matter how many times she disciplined herself to lose weight, her eating and her weight always got out of control.

I worked hard with Joan to make sure she knew exactly the number of calories in every food she was likely to encounter in her busy life. Joan listened carefully and followed my instructions to the letter. She began dropping weight, as she had so many times before. She lost 9 kg (20 lb), and her friends began complimenting her on how great she looked. She was delighted to be back into her 'best' dress size.

But one night, Joan went to a buffet dinner party where the host was offering a delicious chocolate mousse parfait as dessert along with a tray of little cookies. Quickly calculating that the chocolate mouse had four times as many calories as a couple of cookies, Joan bypassed the mousse and took two cookies instead. That was very good caloric thinking. But *historically,* Joan never had eaten just two cookies in her life! If she ate one, she ate 10. And once Joan ate 10 cookies, she could crave a whole bag of cookies the next day – and the next. Once her cookie cravings started again, Joan couldn't resist them. It was *never* true for Joan that one little cookie was 40 calories. One little cookie was just the first of 5,000 calories a month – with no end in sight!

Had Joan bypassed the cookies and eaten a chocolate mousse parfait for dessert instead, she wouldn't have revived the cycle of cravings and bingeing on cookies that was her unique downfall in dieting, and she would not have regained weight. Joan had no *history* of abusing chocolate mousse in her life. If she ate one serving of mousse, she was satisfied. True, that chocolate mousse would have cost her about 300 calories, but it would have been a one-time splurge. She told me she could have even taken a few tastes and left the remainder. Mousse isn't a food that Joan has a history of eating compulsively, nor is it readily available in her day-to-day environment.

But eating compulsively is exactly what Joan did with cookies. By eating just two cookies, she had reactivated her cravings for more. She started eating them on a regular basis, and soon she was regaining her weight. She left a message at my office saying she wanted to take a break from her appointments.

Most diet books will tell you, and even I believed at the time, that 'there are no good foods or bad foods'. I discovered that's a dangerous half-truth. The whole truth is: there are no good foods or bad foods – *there are only good and bad histories with a food.*

It was only after months that Joan returned to my office. She gained back even more weight than she had lost. I suggested we take a look at what happened to her in the months since I'd last seen her and what we might learn together. When I carefully retraced with Joan the path that led to her eating spiralling out of control, we both began to suspect that cookies were a trigger that, time and again, propelled Joan into cycles of cravings and bingeing. It was Joan's life-long history with cookies that was primarily responsible for her repeated failures at weight loss. In addition, once she started overeating cookies, she began to let her guard down with other foods as well.

The difference between an occasional dessert for Joan versus compulsively eating cookies offered a powerful clue to her ability to control her weight. Together, we uncovered the key to perm-anent success at weight control for Joan!

Based on this insight, Joan and I worked out strategies that meant that not only did she not have to give up delicious desserts, but she could even eat satisfying substitutes for cookies that never triggered her cravings. Joan dropped the weight she gained back and has kept it off ever since.

Why It's the Most Essential Strategy

Think historically, not just calorically, is perhaps the most essential strategy of successful weight control. The very instant you begin to think historically, your way of looking at food dramatically changes. You no longer look at the calories in just one biscuit, one roll or one serving of ice cream. Instead, you look at how many biscuits, rolls or scoops of ice cream you *historically* eat, and you can calcu-late how many calories that one biscuit, sweet or scoop of ice cream will ultimately cost you in pounds or kilos. I teach my clients to think in 'calorie units' – how much they would normally eat based on their history – when they look at a food.

I am frequently interviewed on television and radio about weight-loss strategies, and I think it's great when talk show hosts are generous enough to share with their audiences their own difficulties with dieting. One male host talked very candidly with me about how hard it was for him to stay in control of his weight given the hectic life he led. When he paused for a commercial break, I watched him finish up a hefty bag of potato crisps that his assistant had left near his desk. I leaned over and said to him: 'A potato crisp has 500 calories.' He looked at me as if I were crazy! He showed me the nutrition label on the side of the bag: 'A single serving is about 120 calories,' he said. I smiled: 'Do you always finish the bag?' He confessed he did. So I explained: 'If one crisp leads you to eat a whole bag of crisps that size, then one potato crisp is 500 calories – the total number of calories in the bag.' Some months later, I was invited back to his programme. I complimented him on his weight loss, and before I sat down with him at his desk, he showed me a bag of potato crisps – but this time, it was much smaller! 'Now one potato crisp only has 200 calories.' He smiled. 'I'll never order the large bag again.' And I smiled back and said, 'You could be really food smart and buy the *baked* type of potato crisps. You'll save even more!'

Diet Plans: Helping or Hurting You?

Of the many clients who came to me only after failing on a low-carb diet such as Atkins, not a single one of them failed because they couldn't live without pasta or eat a lot of meat. They followed the recommended low-carb menus to the letter, but low-carb diets specifically allow the consumption of high-fat cheeses and peanuts. These clients had a long history of abusing just these foods. Some overate the peanuts consistently. Others would lose control with nibbling on the cheeses. Eventually, these clients stopped losing weight, and before long, they were gaining back the weight they had hoped to lose forever.

I had a very motivated client named Carol who came to me frustrated after failing to lose weight on a well-known weight-control programme. The programme required that its clients buy the company's low-calorie meals in advance each week, including all the snacks allowed in the plan. But the problem for Carol turned out to be her long history of compulsively munching finger foods if they were around her house. Once she brought a week's worth of crackers, sugar-free sweets and pretzels into her home, she'd start picking at them. She'd wind up eating a whole week's worth of snacks in the first 2 days alone.

Carol liked the highly organized structure of the weight programme, and she wanted to succeed with it. So I suggested to Carol that she skip buying the programme's snack foods and instead purchase a single, healthy low-calorie snack each afternoon. (I recommended a yogurt and an apple.) Carol adopted that strategy, and by respecting her unique food history, she began going forward, not backward, on her personal road to being thin, using the meal plans.

GOOD-FOR-YOU FOODS AREN'T ALWAYS GOOD

It's crucial that you realize that very few foods are dietetic or healthy for *you* if *you* have a well-established history of feeding yourself too much of that food. (Although you will find in my diet chapter a number of 'free' foods that have helped make my clients trim.) Newspapers and magazines promote the benefits of eating seven almonds a day, which appears to be a manageable amount of calories in anybody's diet. But I have found that very few people have a history of eating *only* seven almonds and that most people will interpret such well-intentioned advice as a green light to eat handfuls. I've actually never met a man who didn't abuse nuts when eating them by the handful, and I've met many women who share the same problem. The short-sightedness of thinking calorically alone, instead of historically as well, can turn the real cost of seven almonds per day into thousands of excess calories per week!

Studies have shown that people who buy 'reduced-fat' snacks end up consuming more calories than those who buy the higher-fat version. Sometimes that's because more sugar has been added to the products, which triggers compulsive eating, but just as often, it's because people who buy foods labelled low-fat or fat-free think it's 'safe' to binge on them.

The mark of smart people is that once they realize that what they have done in the past is not working for them, they change what they are doing. It's a profound shift in your thinking when you begin to consider your personal history with a piece of food *before* you consider the number of calories in the food. When you know your history, you can predict how you will behave with this food or any food in any and all situations. You won't be misled into violating your food history just because a food is low-calorie or 'healthy'. To shift your thinking, always ask yourself: 'What is my history with this food (or this type of food)?' Then – and only then – look at the calories.

FOLLOWING THIS COMMANDMENT

Remember that people like you gain weight because of predictable eating patterns that involve the same foods, the same behaviours and the same situations.

So how do we discover *your* eating pattern?

When a client first comes to my office, the first thing I do is to explore her food history. I ask her to start by naming any food weaknesses she has. The majority of clients immediately identify either a category of foods, such as sweets, bread products or salty snacks, or specific foods, such as chocolate or salty crisps that trigger them to eat too much of that food. A small minority of clients cite as their eating weakness a particular behaviour, nibbling, or eating because they're bored. A handful of my new clients tell me that they repeatedly lose control of their eating when in certain situations, such as cocktail parties and all-you-can-eat buffets.

While each person has his or her own unique history, all the histories share four common elements that trigger loss of control in eating:

- Trigger foods. People abuse a specific food, whether it is chocolate or bread, or specific types of foods, such as crunchy snacks.
- Trigger behaviours. People repeat a certain specific behaviour that leads to overconsumption, such as skipping meals, picking at food with their fingers or finishing everything on the plate.
- Trigger situations. People repeatedly abuse foods when in certain situations, such as at parties or sports events.
- Trigger times. People abuse food repeatedly at a specific time of the day or week, such as after dinner or while relaxing on Sunday afternoons. Ninety per cent of my clients report few problems with food until the mid-to-late afternoon (typically starting around 3 or 4 p.m.) on into the evening.

I think of an individual's unique pattern of eating as her 'Eating Print'. Just like you have your own unique fingerprint, you have your own unique eating print too. Your eating print is a *dynamic* pattern of foods, behaviours and situations that trigger you to lose control of your eating. It is a repetitive pattern that forms a predictable mosaic of your own personal food weaknesses and eating behaviours. Recognizing your own eating print is one of the single most powerful tools you can use to gain control of your weight.

In psychology, there is an axiom that if you do what you have always done, you will get the result you have always got. You can't do what you have always done and expect to get a different result. That's why knowing your eating print and learning the new strategies in this book can end your cycle of weight gain forever. You can enjoy a wide variety of delicious foods without wearing them – but only if you know your own history!

WHAT ARE YOUR TRIGGER FOODS?

Identifying a trigger food is as simple as it looks. Ask yourself: 'Is this food a weakness of mine? Do I eat one piece (or a single serving) of this food – or 10?' What are the foods that give you the greatest cravings that have also contributed to your greatest weight problems? Your mouth may water at the thought of your sister-in-law's homemade mushroom soup, but soup isn't making you gain weight. Some of you already know your trigger foods under another name – 'comfort foods'. In a recent issue of *More* magazine, a reader wrote in: 'Comfort foods for me are mashed potatoes, cookies and chocolates. But I've finally learned to eat foods that make me feel good *afterward:* fruits, vegetables, fibre and low-fat dairy.' That is a woman who knows her food history and is using smart strategies to deal with it!

The F-Q Principle

One of the hallmarks of a trigger food is that at the beginning of a diet, you usually give it up, out of an intuitive feeling that it will impede your weight control. But once you've lost an amount of weight that pleases you, you feel it's 'safe' to go back to it. At first, you are very focused on not abusing that food. You'll only eat one biscuit or a few potato crisps and walk away from the rest. But it's the beginning of the road backward, although you seldom realize it. If you're thinking calorically, the logic of going back to your old ways proves almost irresistible in the coming days: you had a biscuit or a few crisps and didn't put on any weight, so why not do it again? And again? I call it the F-Q Principle because once the *frequency* starts to increase, invariably the *quantity* will increase as well, until it reaches the amount it was before. And you will gain back the amount of weight you lost before! Thinking calorically, there is nothing wrong with eating one biscuit or a few potato crisps. Yet this behaviour is a bridge back to a pattern of behaviour that may be marked by a long history of overeating, proving once again that history comes before calories!

No More Trigger Foods – Forever?

Once you identify your trigger foods and recognize the role that they are playing in your weight gain, *must* you give them up? Most likely not. Giving up your trigger foods forever is just *one* smart strategy in weight control. Many of my clients use a variety of smart strategies (you will learn many of them in the section on 'boxing in' a food on page 105) that either enable them to keep those foods in their life or switch to substitute foods that they find equally pleasurable.

TRIGGER BEHAVIOURS

New clients sometimes tell me they don't have any food weaknesses at all. They overeat all foods, they say, and they believe that's why they are overweight. What they really mean is that they *finish* all foods. 'Finishing' is a behaviour that triggers overconsumption, just like picking at food with your fingers is another kind of behaviour that triggers overconsumption. Once you know you have a history of being a 'finisher', you can learn strategies to avoid being served fattening foods in a restaurant, so that whatever you finish isn't going to make you heavy. Likewise, once you know you have a history of overconsuming finger foods, even a strategy as simple as always eating your pizza with a knife and fork can stop you from gaining weight. Or when you're at a party, carry a glass of appetite-quenching to-mato juice in one hand and a crunchy crudité in the other. For some people, *the essence of weight control is simply finger control.*

Other kinds of behaviours that lead people to overeat are skipping meals, going food shopping after work, waiting so long to eat that you arrive at a restaurant so starved that you demolish the breadbasket, or overeating at a buffet restaurant. If you have a history of routinely engaging in these types of behaviours, you will find that the Fourth Thin Commandment, Structure Gives Control, is filled with strategies that address precisely these issues (see page 74).

TRIGGER TIMES AND SITUATIONS

One of the most predictable and fascinating things about dieters is that if they gain back the weight they lost, they will not only do it with the same foods and the same behaviours, they will do it in the *same places* and at the *same times* that they gained that weight the first time around. In-store bakeries, set-menu restaurants and sweet shops trigger overconsumption for many people. It can also be that a certain day of the week, like having long hours of free time on a weekend afternoon, triggers some people to overeat. Many of my clients report that they have no problems with food until the hours between 4 o'clock and 5 o'clock every afternoon – those are the times that they fall prey to the foods and eating behaviours that cause them to gain weight.

To help raise your level of awareness, I've ranked the top three problem-eating times in order of frequency:

1. Later afternoon

2. Evenings – while waiting for dinner

3. Weekend afternoons at home

Very few people tend to overeat in the morning or the early part of the day.

THE PREDICTABILITY OF YOUR EATING BEHAVIOUR

If you see that never in your entire lifetime have you been able to eat just seven nuts, or skip breakfast without gorging later, nor can

How Does This Commandment Make You a Weight-Control Winner?

1. It predicts your behaviour in advance with any food you have eaten in your life.
2. It predicts the time of the day when you are most likely to be vulnerable to overeating.
3. It predicts the types of situations that are most associated with losses of control.
4. It helps you evaluate food in a new way – not just in terms of counting calories and carbohydrates, but in terms of how any food affects your behaviour, appetite, control and success at dieting.
5. It helps you set up boundaries that come out of your own unique life history and break through the feelings of deprivation that haunt your own life.
6. It shifts your thinking from being 'good' or 'bad' to thinking in terms of 'what works or doesn't work for me'.

you stay away from chips on a weekend, you can predict with certainty that you will gain weight by continuing down that path. Or you can take control of your life by learning the strategies that will change your history and create a happier future for yourself.

Predictability is the highest goal of all science. Knowing your own history hands you the key to the *most* scientific approach you will ever find to losing weight. When you can predict in advance your responses to food based on your history and use strategy accordingly, you stop being a victim who marches blindly through the world of food, tripping over the same potholes again and again.

When you understand your own food history, you finally understand that it's not the whole world of food against you. Nor is the whole world of dieting against you. When you think in terms of your own unique food history *first*, you see that the problem may never have been with you at all, but with the food itself.

Each person is a living textbook of one. There is tremendous biological variability in our species, so what may be completely unappealing to someone else may drive you into an eating frenzy.

The Third Thin Commandment:
The Problem May Be in the Food, Not in You

COMMANDMENT ESSENTIALS

- Kill appetite cravings with a sweet protein shake when fruit won't do the trick.
- Don't skip meals or go too long without eating.
- Eat a protein or a protein with high fibre for breakfast.
- Substitute pickles or V-8 juice with a dash of Tabasco when tempted to indulge in sweets.
- Never try to correct for overeating by skipping meals the following day.
- Be aware of SAD cold-weather eating.
- Keep your home a 'junk food–free' zone.

THE FOLLOWING SCENARIO IS as predictable as a Hollywood action movie. Call it *Diet Terminator.* You commit yourself to losing weight. You have all the best intentions of sticking with a diet and actually do so for a while. Until…a tray of pastries shoots you a tempting glance. Or you inhale the riveting aroma of a pizza bubbling in a brick oven, or perhaps you'll just have a few nuts from that bowl of cashews. The next thing you know, you're sitting in a bloated stupor, wondering how a tiny bite of food led to eating so much more than you ever intended. You call yourself weak and undisciplined and think that you have no willpower. You might even suspect that you have an eating disorder.

You may be dead wrong. A whole new field of scientific research is emerging that may explain why you have failed so often in your dieting. This research is exploring how the foods you eat today may change the chemistry of your brain in such a way as to increase your appetite and cravings for these and other foods – even without you being aware that this process is taking place.

Just as the first chapter discussed changing your thinking, so this chapter will address your physical makeup and its influence on your food choices and teach you how to be a winner at weight control. You'll learn about the physiological basis of appetite, why you may be having recurring problems controlling certain foods, and how to make your body work *for* you, not against you. Using this knowledge, you'll be able to reduce or even eliminate your cravings for certain foods and, for the first time, have the power to take control of foods that have sabotaged your weight loss again and again.

These new studies may even change your own perception of yourself as a person lacking willpower, as someone who has never succeeded on a diet because you lacked backbone.

Thanks to the latest scientific research, we've learned that while *weight control is primarily about balancing calories in and calories out, appetite and craving control is about the types of foods you eat and how they interact with your body's genetic and chemical hardwiring. In short, the problem may be in the food, not in you.*

In fact, what may surprise you is that your eating behaviour and the very foods you choose for breakfast, lunch and dinner today may be influenced by the interaction of the food with your genetics and neurochemistry. This process is going on without your knowing it, which is why you may overconsume these foods without intending to. (Remember those promises to yourself: 'I'll have just one'?) It may also explain why you keep regaining the same weight with the same foods, despite the best of intentions.

Now, as science is revealing that the problem may be in the food, not in you, the good news is that even if you have genetic sensitivities to certain foods, all you need are the right strategies to manage them. And for those of you who prefer to get a certain food out of your life completely, I'll provide the powerful tools to not only make it possible, but easy.

So if you have an uncontrollable craving for a particular food that unleashes a furious eating bender, you'll be relieved to discover that this urge doesn't prove that you are a spineless mess with a weak character. Or that you can't succeed at weight control. All it proves is that you are human – and you need strategy.

DOES OUR DNA RULE OUR APPETITES?

Genes exert a tremendous influence over both our biology – they give us such things as red hair and blue eyes – and our behaviour. *But up to now, we've never realized genes' influence over our eating habits, our appetites and the type of diet we should follow – and even whether or not we'll succeed on that diet.*

Your genes may send powerful, unconscious messages that impel you to, say, make a beeline for the pastry aisle or to accumulate more than a few extra pounds of fat. While these urges can cause us grief, they have a sound basis in evolution. As Terry Burnham and Jay Phelan write in their book *Mean Genes*, 'Our ancestors lived off the land by hunting animals and gathering plants... Just staying alive required lots of energy – energy that could be found only in food...' What kept our ancestors going in a tough, physically demanding world? Hunger. Our ancestors needed to stay hungry day and night; their only goal was storing enough food to keep them alive during the inevitable lean times. And they sought not just any kind of food, but calorically dense, fatty foods. But while this kind of gluttony was necessary for survival in the Neolithic African bush, in our ultra-convenient, sedentary society of plenty, it only leads to expanding waistlines.

Scientists have clearly established that for many of us, our genes play a large role in controlling our weight, as confirmed by the following discoveries:

- Hereditary factors can impact our appetites.
- Genes may regulate how efficiently we convert food into energy, which can affect our weight.
- In 2002, scientists discovered a gene, HOB1, that they promptly labelled the 'fat gene'. They've also identified from

8 to 30 other genes that may contribute to obesity by inhibiting the body's metabolism.
- Researchers at the Monell Chemical Senses Center are working on discovering a 'sweet tooth' gene that would locate a person's vulnerability to sweet cravings.

JUMP-START YOUR APPETITE

Hormones are complex molecules produced by the endocrine glands that manage many bodily functions and processes. One of the most important hormones for appetite is insulin, the 'hunger hormone', which the body uses to process glucose (sugar) and mediate our cravings for fat and carbohydrates. The level of insulin also influences the storage of calories as fat and even the degree to which we may be able to lose weight on a particular diet.

When blood glucose rises, your pancreas produces insulin, which converts the excess glucose to glycogen (glucose stored in the liver) or fat. When your blood glucose dips too low, and you don't replenish it by eating, your body siphons glycogen. Normally, this process is neatly balanced, and insulin and other hormones help you maintain a stable body weight.

However, your diet can shatter this equilibrium. If you consume large amounts of refined simple carbohydrates, *and* you're significantly overweight (especially with abdominal fat), you can cause the pancreas to become a superproductive insulin factory, creating the condition known as 'insulin resistance'.

A person with insulin resistance has to produce more insulin to reduce his blood glucose to normal levels, according to Dr Walter Futterweit, one of America's leading endocrinologists. The increasing amounts of insulin lead to hyperinsulinism – too much of it in the body. All that insulin can increase your appetite and lead to fatigue, lack of concentration, shakiness, sweats and an excessive lowering of blood sugar called reactive hypoglycaemia. At this point, you may try to get relief by taking in more simple carbohydrates, which only causes more insulin production in a damaging cycle. It's important to note that even if you are not insulin resistant, but you go too long without eating, you can create a state of induced reactive hypoglycemia with the same cravings and symptoms.

In working with thousands of clients, it has been my observation that a large number of them have had insulin cravings for carbohydrates, and giving them a diet that includes such foods as biscuits, pasta, bagels and sugary breakfast cereals may actually increase their cravings for more and lead to a heightened appetite throughout the day.

A study conducted by Peter Havel of the University of California and Michael Schwartz of the University of Washington also revealed that *over time*, a diet high in fat and fructose (a sugar frequently found in healthy products such as many bran muffins and baked goods) may affect insulin levels and increase appetite. *The food itself is actually increasing the person's cravings, appetite and hunger level.* What's worse, Schwartz says, is that the brain loses its ability to respond to insulin as a person gets fatter and/or when fat is more than 30 per cent of the person's diet. Under these conditions, tissues also may become insensitive to insulin, and carbohydrate cravings are intensified.

In June 2004, a study by researchers at the Monell Center in Philadelphia also suggested that overconsumption of fructose seems to alter appetite-regulating hormones in a way that stimulates overeating.

People in the study who ate a meal followed by a drink containing the same amount of fructose as that found in two cans of soda showed relatively low levels of insulin and leptin (another hormone that signals to people that they are full), and higher levels of ghrelin, a hormone that stimulates eating.

According to Sarah Leibowitz, PhD, a professor at the Rockefeller University laboratory of behavioural neuroscience in New York City and one of the pre-eminent researchers of the physiological basis of eating behaviour and weight, hormones also have been known to increase appetite and craving for sweets or meat in women with premenstrual syndrome. The hormones are acting under the evolutionary pressure of genes; it's nature's way of telling a woman that she needs extra fat calories if she wants to produce a child.

Finally, stress – whether physical or psychological – also can wreak havoc with weight control by releasing the so-called stress hormones – adrenalin, corticotrophin-releasing hormone (CRH) and cortisol – to meet what the body perceives as an emergency.

Carb Cravings and Why You Can't Lose Weight

Millions of women may not be aware that they have a condition that is making it difficult for them to lose weight and fuelling cravings for carbohydrates, especially sweets.

Polycystic ovary syndrome (PCOS) is a serious condition that affects 5 to 9 per cent of the women of reproductive age; half of these women are overweight.

Women with PCOS suffer irregular menstrual cycles during adolescence; their symptoms may also include acne and other skin conditions, irregular hair growth or thinning hair.

From 30 to 40 per cent of obese patients with PCOS, at the time they're first seen by a doctor, already have an abnormally high tolerance for sugar and an increased frequency of type 2 diabetes, says Dr Walter Futterweit, one of the world's premier authorities on PCOS, whose groundbreaking studies have helped identify the mechanisms of PCOS.

Both high insulin levels and insulin resistance are very common in this syndrome, which explains why many women with PCOS have increased cravings for sweets. And after they eat biscuits, sweets, sweet juices or other carbohydrates such as pasta, they often develop other symptoms such as sleepiness, lack of concentration and occasional shakiness and sweatiness. In addition, diets with even a limited amount of these foods may make it extremely difficult for them to lose weight – even though they may be restricting calories. If you suspect that you have this condition, you should consult your doctor. (You can also find more information at www.verity-pcos.org.uk or www.posaa.asn.au.)

Women with PCOS have trouble losing weight while their diet contains high or even medium amounts of carbohydrates. Dr Futterweit advises women with PCOS to go on a low-carbohydrate diet and eat small meals throughout the day, always including some protein when they eat carbohydrates. An eating plan such as one given in this book, based on low-fat protein, nonstarchy vegetables, healthy monounsaturated oil found in seafood and fish, poultry, eggs and low-fat dairy, plus limited amounts of fruit, would be ideal for women with this condition. If you switch to this way of eating, you should find a decrease in your craving for carbohydrates and an increase in your weight loss.

High amounts of cortisol may cause deposits of fat around the midsection. Stress also depletes your body's glycogen fuel reserves. And the longer and more intense the stress, the lower your blood sugar will dip, which often leads to carbohydrate cravings. *Yes, your stress may make you hungry and cause you to store more fat.*

And, of course, one of our favourite ways to relieve stress is by reaching for the nearest chocolate bar or biscuit, which leads to higher insulin levels and carb cravings in what can be a destructive loop of perpetual craving and eating.

So as you can see, the hormones in your blood and the chemicals in your brain perform a delicate balancing act that requires smart food strategies to avoid trouble. And you'll learn some very creative strategies to master stress and lose weight comfortably in the Fifth Commandment, Separate Mood from Food (see page 90).

CAN YOU BE ADDICTED TO CAKE?

Dopamine is a neurotransmitter – a molecule that sends messages from one neuron in the brain to another – produced by an enzymatic pathway in the brain. It's been called the 'feel-good molecule'. It creates pleasurable sensations in your brain every time you have sex, hear your favourite music, dig into an ice cream sundae or (unfortunately) use cocaine. Scientists have isolated it as a key to understanding drug and alcohol addiction.

While drugs such as alcohol, cocaine and opiates seem to boost the release of dopamine and other neurochemicals involved in the change in thought and behaviour that characterize addictive states, recent findings suggest that these same neurochemicals may be involved even when we form dependencies on such things as coffee, cake or gambling. And scientists such as Harvard psychiatry professor Hans Breiter have discovered through magnetic resonance imaging that the same brain centres that are activated during the ecstasy of drug use also do so in compulsive gamblers on a 'high'.

This suggests the conclusion that not only drug use but any recurring activity that triggers dopamine release, such as eating certain foods, can reshape the brain in important ways – ways that compel you to keep repeating that action and that make 'Just saying no' much more difficult. Scientists call this neuroadaptation, and it could at least partially explain why you can't stop yourself from wolfing down those chocolate-covered raisins. (This is not to say that dopamine is the only chemical involved in the thought processes of drug abusers or addictive-like behaviours.)

While I'm careful not to overuse the term 'addiction', a leading expert has pointed out, 'if you look at all addictions from tobacco to heroin, there's only one clear statement that applies to all of them: uncontrolled use despite negative consequences'. Our present epidemic of obesity and compulsive eating may share some remarkable similarities of behaviour and neurobiology with that observation.

It's important to realize when we speak about an addictive or addictive-like relationship with a substance or a food that the research holds out the hope that this relationship can be reversed through learning.

Journalist Madeleine Nash, in a very revealing article on addictive behaviour in *Time* magazine, came to an important insight after reviewing the studies and various modalities of treatment: 'One of the most hopeful messages coming out of current research is that the biochemical abnormalities associated with addiction can be reversed through learning. For that reason, all sorts of psychological interventions, ranging from psychotherapy to 12-Step programming, can and do help. Cognitive therapy, which seeks to supply people with coping skills – exercising after work instead of going to a bar – appears to hold particular promise. After just 10 weeks of therapy, before-and-after PET-scans [positive emission tomography] of the brain suggest that some patients suffering from obsessive-compulsive disorders manage to resculpt not only their behavior but also activity patterns in their brain.' Having developed strategies for thousands of compulsive eaters that helped them to lose the cravings and the interest in foods they had been out of control with for decades, I can only say, 'Amen!'

Perhaps most significant in this analysis is that teaching people coping skills not only changes their behaviour but may change the brain activity that underlies it. That's why strategy is so critical in managing certain types of foods.

In the end, you should listen to your body when it comes to food. Just because your symptoms may not meet someone's textbook definition of addiction doesn't mean they don't exist. And as we shall see now, there is another factor that may impel you to act like an addict by craving more and more carbohydrates or fuelling your appetite and a cycle of compulsive overeating.

NEUROPEPTIDE Y: THE MISSING LINK IN CRAVING CONTROL?

Up to now, we've been talking about genetics and environmental and neurochemical factors and their instinctive influence on your eating. However, *to a large degree, your response to food is primarily in your own hands.* A classic example of how your behaviour influences the control of appetite and the success of your diet is the case of neuropeptide Y.

Have you ever noticed that if you've gone a number of hours without eating, skipped meals or just eaten too little, by a certain part of the day, usually the late afternoon, your appetite starts to rev up? Well, so does almost everybody else's. In a recent survey, 98 per cent of participants in a weight-control programme said they tend to overeat at the same time each day.

Why is this? Dr Sarah Leibowitz's studies suggest that this clockwork craving may be caused by surging levels of a protein known as neuropeptide Y, which may contribute to 'a stimulatory effect on food intake, particularly carbohydrate ingestion'.

While Dr Leibowitz's groundbreaking research focuses on animals, Dr C. Wayne Calloway, an endocrinologist at George Washington University in Washington, D.C., is a clinician working with weight-control patients. He explained to *Allure* magazine, 'If the body has been deprived of sufficient calories during the day, the levels of metabolic regulator neuropeptide Y will rise once one starts eating. This leads to greater cravings for food, especially carbohydrates…At that point, it's hard to resist the body's chemical signals to consume. You turn into an eating automaton, without being aware of it. If you think you're an intelligent, responsible person, it's spooky how little control you have over this.'

Neuropeptide Y is so powerful that it imprints whatever you eat on an empty stomach on your brain's craving control centre. And those foods – especially simple carbs such as sweets, refined flour products and baked goods – deactivate your appetite-control mechanism and may ignite increased cravings for more and more, even though you intend to 'have just a little'.

It's very critical to understand the interaction of all these processes, which combine to make so many people feel like they lack willpower to fight their seemingly insatiable appetite. The truth is that if you've gone beyond a few hours without eating, then having a biscuit, that biscuit, instead of satisfying you, becomes a turbocharged appetite stimulant causing you to overeat. This can be true even if you've never craved biscuits before, a fact proven by a 1990 study at University College, London, in which subjects who were indifferent to chocolate but ate it on an empty stomach ended up craving it.

Can a Craving Be Unlearned?

The same British researchers who discovered that people who didn't particularly care for chocolate developed cravings for it when they ate it on an empty stomach may also have found a way to 'unlearn' a craving. Chocolate junkies who ate half a bar immediately after lunch and half a bar immediately after dinner for 2 weeks lost their craving for chocolate. The key to losing the craving appears to rest in (1) eating it when you're not hungry and the stomach is full (this is critical), and (2) 'flooding yourself' with the taste of the food by having it repeatedly (i.e., twice a day) for 2 weeks. Apparently, no matter how much you like a food or how much it has retarded your progress at weight control, you may be able to extinguish your cravings for it. You can use this same technique to eliminate or reduce cravings for foods that have held back your progress at weight control. But beware the reverse can also be true; if you eat it on an empty stomach or in place of a meal, you can increase your cravings!

Food Memories and the 'Proust Factor'

In Marcel Proust's classic, *In Search of Lost Time*, the autobiographical protagonist, Marcel, bites into a biscuit called a madeleine, which generates a memory of when he first sampled the biscuit as a child. From this reminiscence, a tidal wave of other memories and associations washes over him (enough to fill seven volumes!).

Proust's 'appetite memory' led to the creation of a literary masterpiece. But this kind of powerful recollection can also create cravings for certain foods. It could be years since you tasted that special biscuit, but one bite would bring back the longing for its sugary chewiness. This thought is called an 'emotional memory'.

Along with these memories, cravings can be triggered by the visual stimulus of food and its aroma, which produce neurochemical changes in the brain that ignite its appetite craving centre. Numerous studies show that the more foods you see and keep around your home, the more you eat and the more frequently you eat – even if you're not hungry. And let's face it, in our culture, food is everywhere – all around your house, in restaurants, takeaways and supermarkets, and buffets in conference rooms and meetings. Kelly Brownell, a professor of psychology at Yale, has wisely described this as a 'toxic food environment' – and your own home may be the most toxic.

Whether it's genes or behaviour, nature or nurture, eating behaviour for many of us becomes habitual very quickly. I call it the power of 'just one bite'. For example, many of my clients who eat in restaurants make a decision not to touch the breadbasket and go many weeks, months or even years abstaining. The breadbasket stops being a major source of temptation, and they may even stop being aware of it. Then they're tempted one evening by the aroma of a freshly baked roll in a fine restaurant. One leads to two, and soon enough, they've gone back to ransacking the breadbasket. First, they eat it out of preference; then they eat it out of habit.

For Proust, an emotional memory was a bridge back to the past of his idealized childhood, but for you, it could be a bridge back to a time or place when you abused foods – a past you'd rather not revisit.

TASTE BUDS: A CRITICAL KEY TO APPETITE CONTROL

There is yet another reason why so many of my clients may be able to have 'just one' biscuit, then stop eating, while a second person can go from one biscuit to 10 in no time flat. It has to do with the number of taste buds, the groups of cells on our tongue that distinguish between sweet and bitter, salty and creamy. So often my clients have asked me why they don't have the willpower of their spouse to have just one biscuit. I look at them and smile and say,

'He may not have more willpower than you, but he may have more taste buds on his tongue.'

Linda Bartoshuk, a professor of the Yale University School of Medicine, has conducted years of pioneering research on taste buds that I believe will have strong implications for weight control. She has discovered that some people may have a few hundred taste buds on their tongue, while others have tens of thousands. The former group, called 'nontasters', has a high tolerance for and often desire fatty, salty and bitter foods, which cause them to indulge in them more frequently.

On the other hand, the 'supertasters' have highly sensitive palates. Food 'floods' over them; sweet tastes a lot sweeter and fat a lot fatter. They're easily repulsed by bitter flavours. In the middle are 'medium tasters'.

The supertasters are perfectly sated by one biscuit. But by the time the nontasters reach their point of satiety, they've taken in so much sugar, flour and/or fat that it's affecting their neurochemistry and setting in motion overconsumption or binge eating.

Taste bud differential may also explain why some people can't have 'just one' potato crisp for 'crunch' – and why salt may serve as a major appetite trigger. You see, if the potato crisp was soggy, they would have no trouble stopping at one. (To find out what kind of taster you are, see 'Test Your Taste Buds' below.)

Test Your Taste Buds

There are two simple ways for you to determine what kind of taster you are. (1) Put some saccharine on the tip of your tongue. If you taste only sweetness, you are probably a nontaster. But if you taste sweetness and bitterness, you're most likely a medium taster. If the saccharine tastes extremely bitter, you're a supertaster.

(2) Put some blue food colouring on the tip of your tongue. If you're a supertaster, your tongue will look covered in pink dots, called fungiform papillae. If you're a medium taster, you'll see half white dots and half pink dots. If your tongue looks more polka-dotted, with many fewer pink dots, you're probably a nontaster.

This research is only in its infancy, and among other things, we're learning that gender and race seem to have an effect on the number of taste buds you have. Thirty-five per cent of women are more likely to be supertasters, as opposed to only 15 per cent of men. And more Asians than Caucasians are supertasters, which means they often find sugary foods cloying and prefer less sweet desserts. That's why none of my clients has ever gone to a Japanese or Chinese restaurant in a desperate search for a dessert!

However, the critical point is that an inborn, genetic predisposition influences how powerfully we respond to the taste and texture of food. What is sickeningly sweet to one person may prove to be the ultimate treat to another. A second crucial point is made by Valerie Duffy, PhD, an assistant professor of dietetics at the University of Connecticut: 'People tend to look at someone who's overweight and say, "He has no willpower" or "Why can't she just walk away from food?" When the truth is that it just may be easier for some people to turn down certain foods because of their taste bud structure.' As Dr Duffy implies, *this is not about willpower*, as illustrated by the following anecdote:

The work of Drs Bartoshuk, Duffy and other taste bud researchers suggests that (1) people may live 'in different worlds of taste'; (2) this biological variability influences how much you will typically eat of a certain food, i.e., whether you can consume it moderately or abuse it; (3) why some people are 'finishers' of certain foods – they'll always feel compelled to finish a dessert while others are satisfied with a taste; and most important, (4) your taste preferences may influence what types of food you buy in the supermarket or order in a restaurant and how much you weigh.

Taste bud research also may help us understand that the dynamics of compulsive eating for many may be more accurately explained in terms of physiology rather than psychopathology. These studies, along with the neuropeptide Y phenomenon, clearly lend credence to one of the favourite adages I have imparted to my clients – 'You don't have to be crazy to be crazy about a cookie!' A genetic sensitivity to sugar or salt plus very few taste buds, which typically leads to overconsuming, can easily become a dangerous mix. Since nontasters may need to consume a large quantity of sugary or salty foods to feel satisfied, they trigger a tremendous amount of insulin, the hunger hormone. So instead of eating just one or two cookies, they find themselves finishing the whole packet.

The good news is that with strategy, you'll soon *learn to handle your physiology and still keep your favourite foods in your life – and remain your favourite size!*

HOW WILL THIS COMMANDMENT HELP YOU?

What can we learn from the scientific research discussed in this chapter to increase success at weight control and to make it easy? By understanding how the timing of your eating and the types of foods you eat affect your appetite, you have the knowledge to change your attitude and then your behaviour. Here's what this commandment provides:

• It relieves guilt by helping you understand that any binges or compulsive overeating may not be due to personal weakness but may instead be a reflection of powerful, complex biochemical forces and how they interact with certain foods you select – and at what time of the day and under what conditions you eat them.

If You Sleep Too Little, You Could Eat Too Much

Sometimes my clients tell me they've been hungry all week. In helping them figure out the reason for their hunger, I ask them if they've been sleeping properly. They often look surprised at this question – but they shouldn't be. Sleep deprivation is known to jump-start your appetite, particularly carbohydrate cravings. Studies have demonstrated that depriving both lab animals and humans of sleep increased both their appetites and food consumption. One study of college students found that getting only 2½ hours of sleep for 3 nights in a row and interrupting their sleep on 3 other nights greatly increased their appetite. Another study of young men who were deprived of REM sleep demonstrated a marked increase in appetite.

• It helps you realize that all your previous failures at weight control may have had very little to do with a lack of willpower, but instead a lack of strategy to deal with your genetic sensitivity.

• It points the way to possible solutions – such as food shopping and dining strategies that help you control salty or sweet foods or foods with creamy and/or crunchy textures – if you think you're bingeing or you think you have an eating disorder.

• It describes the types of foods that won't trigger overconsumption and warns you of the ones that will.

• It explains why, if you haven't eaten for several hours, and you then eat simple carbohydrates such as low-fibre crackers, sweets, biscuits and crisps, you may find yourself getting increasingly hungry and overconsuming for the next few hours.

• It helps to explain why, if you can't stop to eat during the day (or if you eat too little), you may find you can't stop eating at night.

• It helps you understand which foods you're hypersensitive to and why your family or friends can have a taste of this food, but if *you* start, you feel a compulsive need for more and more.

• It helps you understand that you may live in a different world of taste and that you should adjust your food choices to succeed in that world.

• It reveals research suggesting that breakfasts consisting of simple carbs such as instant oats, low-fibre sugary breakfast cereals, croissants or bagels, may actually trigger appetite and lead to increased consumption for the entire day.

• It changes our notion of what makes a good snack for weight and appetite control. Most weight programmes allow you a snack in between meals. Make certain this snack is one that does not trigger appetite and cravings.

• It suggests that diets recommended by certain weight-control programmes, which ignore your food history and don't take into account your genetic sensitivity to certain foods or snacks or provide any strategies to deal with them, may actually be causing you to have cravings, lose control and fail at the very diet they are trying to help you follow.

In subsequent chapters, I'll present a wide range of successful strategies to help you lose weight and keep it off. However, if you abandon these strategies and go head to head with your physiology, the likelihood that you'll succeed is very small.

Tips for Ending Your Cravings

One of the most powerful observations we can draw from the neuropeptide Y and British craving research is that we have the power to either end or diminish our cravings or to fuel them to an unmanageable level, often unknowingly. A lot of the people who feel that they're doomed to fail because of their cravings for high-caloric foods or foods they continually abuse can now use the following strategies to end the cravings.

- Don't skip meals or go too long without eating.
- Start your day with a breakfast that doesn't trigger hunger or increased carbohydrate cravings later on.
- Eat a protein or a protein with high fibre for breakfast (which is the best breakfast for many people), such as yogurt with fresh fruit sprinkled with a few tablespoons of high-fibre cereal such as All-Bran. Alternately, try an omelette (or egg-white omelette) with fresh vegetables and/or low-fat cheese, or try my recommended GG Scandinavian Bran Crispbread (the only high-fibre cracker I've ever found that has a sum total of zero net carbs and a mere 18 calories) – literally a crunchy carb without carbs – with Laughing Cow Light cheese wedges melted over it.
- If you like to eat cereal for breakfast, I've found that a high-fibre cereal with protein, such as All-Bran with skimmed milk, doesn't stimulate appetite later in the day for most people. Be careful to measure out a single serving. (Most people typically pour an indiscriminate amount into their breakfast bowl that may be three or four times the calories on the box plus the extra milk calories.)
- Make protein or a protein combined with a high-fibre food your snack of choice for that late-afternoon or early evening period. (See Part 2, starting on page 195, for recommendations.)
- Don't be tricked by many so-called health-food snacks such as cereal or 'breakfast' bars, which often have single-digit grams of fibre and double-digit grams of sugar or fructose.
- Try a heavy, liquid sweet, such as a low-cal hot chocolate or sweet protein shake, to kill appetite and cravings safely when fruit

is unsatisfying or actually increases cravings/appetite in the later afternoon (when neuropeptide Y is rising).

• Be aware of SAD cold-weather eating. *Those suffering from SAD who experience increased appetite cravings or cravings for carbohydrates can still find success at weight control during the winter months with healthy carbohydrates that are sweet such as baked sweet potatoes or the previously suggested bran crackers sweetened with a little low-carb preserve.* Whether or not you suffer from SAD, the winter may bring a shift in food preferences toward hot and heavy meals.

• Detoxify your home food environment. This starts at your supermarket and ends in your refrigerator and kitchen cupboards. Strive to set up an eating and living environment conducive to healthy living.

• Limit post-exercise snacks or meals to foods high in protein and/or fibre or a high-fibre low-carbohydrate variety.

• Never try to correct an overeating/bingeing error by skipping meals or eating miniscule amounts of food the next day. Doing so will only fuel further overconsumption by the end of the day. Instead, eat full meals that offer large volume but low calories such as seafood and low-fat omelettes. A less-satisfactory alternative would be low-fat meats such as turkey or pork.

• Never go hungry to restaurants or events such as meetings or conferences where food is available. That's because the first thing you may be confronted with is a breadbasket, baked goods or nibbles, which will trigger the neuropeptide Y storm and, later, hunger and cravings.

• Realize that seeing and smelling foods you love – or even reading about them – can trip your appetite alarm, even when you're not hungry.

• Be aware that as a nontaster (which means that you need large amounts of sweets and/or salt to fill you up), eating a small amount may be very difficult for you physiologically. *Correct for this by buying a single-size serving at the supermarket, or order it in a controlled setting such as a restaurant, where you'll be given a single serving.*

Once again, in evaluating these strategies, use your own food history as the ultimate litmus test of how your body will respond to the food in question and the need for control strategies.

The taste bud and neuropeptide Y research can also be used in reverse, to encourage consumption of healthy foods you do not like. Here's what to do to help dupe your tongue into savouring foods that ordinarily repel it:

• Add a small amount of salt or spice when cooking pungent vegetables such as cauliflower and brussels sprouts, or blanch them in salt for a couple of minutes before you eat them. Salt blocks bitterness. To avoid excess salt, try a splash of balsamic vinegar, lemon juice, or low-sodium soy sauce.

• Top those hard-to-swallow veggies with some sautéed bread crumbs or a little crumbly light cheese. A little light feta is a good option.

• Add 2 tablespoons of a light or reduced-fat cheese or the same amount of raisins to your salad.

• Sprinkle a pinch of sugar or artificial sweetener on your grapefruit or other tart fruits. This strategy will also work for a tub of natural yogurt, so you can avoid the high sugar of many low-fat or fat-free yogurts.

GENES IMPEL; THEY DON'T COMPEL

One of the greatest rewards and passions of my work has not only been to lift the pain of pounds of fat and a lifelong history of failure in thousands of individuals, but most of all to end years of guilt and self-blame and rid people of the notion that they have a psychopathology, eating disorder, or lack the strength of willpower. When I explain the implications of this research to my clients, a light goes on in their psyche and they immediately understand what had been inexplicable for years.

The research on genes points clearly to the importance of smart food strategies. It has implications for appetite and weight control, shopping, how you display food and where you keep it in your house. However, remember one thing: *genes impel; they don't compel.* And with smart food-management strategies, you can take control of the food, your genetic influence and your weight. This chapter doesn't just explain why you may have found yourself repeatedly gaining back the same weight with the same foods. It sets the stage for appreciating the importance of the strategies to come, such as boxing it in, which will teach you to keep your favourite foods in your life and be in control of them – rather than letting them control you.

(Individuals in psychotherapy for psychological issues related to compulsive eating should not discontinue their therapy, but should bring this research to the attention of their therapist, so that this therapy may yield a more complete and permanent result.)

Lastly, it has great implications for your maintenance programme, because even once you lose the weight, that doesn't mean you've lost the genetic sensitivity to the sight, taste and smell of your trigger foods. And if you get sloppy about the structure of your eating habits and strategies, as many people do once they have lost the weight, you'll end up out of control again. More people have ended up fat again and again not because they're failing, but because they are failing to plan. When reading this chapter, you realize how one commandment builds on the other: that the structure of your eating habits as well as the types of food, the timing and the situation (whether you eat certain types of food on an empty stomach or a full stomach) are critical variables that may either have never been discussed before or were simply ignored. They may be the foundation stone for determining your success at weight control and whether you'll be constantly hungry and have cravings or find it easy to succeed.

We can't change our basic genetic response to food, but we can alter it powerfully through strategy. Whether we control it or it controls us is up to us, through the power of these techniques.

One of the most powerful lessons I have learned from the failures of thousands of people at weight control is *not* that those who fail have no willpower. It is that they had no structure for their eating.

The Fourth Thin Commandment:
Structure Gives Control

COMMANDMENT ESSENTIALS

- Eat a snack with protein and fibre between 3 and 5 p.m.
- Always take your own healthy snack to a meeting.
- Put together a 'ThinPack', and never leave home without it.
- Do your food shopping right after breakfast or right after eating.
- Stay away from food 'minis', such as mini-muffins, mini-doughnuts and mini-cookies.
- At buffets and cocktail parties, use the smallest plate available to serve yourself.

HAVE YOU EVER WONDERED WHY everybody swears by the latest diet, and you often end up knowing quite a few people who lose weight on it? You may have tried a few different diets yourself and found that each time you started a new one, you began dropping weight too.

What is the key ingredient that makes any diet work at the beginning, even though they are so different in their menu plans?

What all diets have in common is *structure*. They all achieve weight loss because they give you a blueprint for eating. Is there a diet in the world that doesn't tell you to eat three good meals every day plus a healthy snack in the afternoon? That *structure* reins in eating behaviour that has been out of control.

So why do the vast majority of people who lose weight on diets fail to maintain that weight loss?

When dieters are taught to focus exclusively on calories and carbs, they don't see anything wrong with fiddling with the structure of their diets. They are led to believe that all that really matters is the 'calorie budget'. My client Paula was doing beautifully on her diet until she went back to skipping breakfast because that was her history from childhood. She began 'making up' the calories with pizza for lunch. Similarly, Sandra eliminated her mid-afternoon snack, figuring she'd 'lay away' those 200 calories and 'spend' them on dessert after dinner. Ed started his diet by studying low-calorie menu plans and prepared all his meals at home. Three weeks later, when he'd lost enough weight to wear his tennis shorts without embarrassment, he went back to eating at his favourite all-you-can-eat buffet restaurant, figuring he could just as easily find low-calorie foods for his plate so it wouldn't be a problem.

The standard diets actually encourage people to play around with the diet, yet they fail to teach you the right *strategies* to keep you from returning to out-of-school eating. They don't help you see *the critical connection between structure and weight control.*

THE WALL STREET EATING SYNDROME

I discovered the critical relationship between structure and weight control by accident. Since I do my work in New York City, I have an unusually large number of clients who work on Wall Street. The lives of these busy people are characterized by extraordinary focus and accomplishment. Many have reached the top of one of the toughest professions in the world, and they did it in one of the toughest cities in the world. Yet each one of them had a long history of failure on weight programmes – so plainly, the problem wasn't willpower!

Clark was the model of the successful Wall Street executive when he became my client: he had a top-floor office overlooking the Statue of Liberty and a wonderful home in the suburbs. He also epitomized the collection of eating habits I now call the Wall Street Eating Syndrome: breakfast was a doughnut or a bagel with coffee that Clark grabbed at the train station on his way to work; when he was running late, he missed breakfast completely. Lunch for Clark was whatever was quickest. Sometimes he'd just grab a bag of cashews or a mere 90-calorie pot of yogurt he 'borrowed' from his assistant. Then if he felt hungry because of having eaten too little, he would nibble on whatever snack foods were around the office or in the conference rooms. Most days, Clark waited until the New York Stock Market closed at 3 p.m. to eat his lunch, then he bolted down a sandwich or whatever food he could find in the company kitchen on his floor. Some days, he just kept picking on whatever was left over from meetings in the conference room.

Clark often had to entertain business associates after work, and if he was sitting at a bar having a beer, he'd eat all the crunchy things in the snack bowl. If he met people at a restaurant, he'd virtually demolish the breadbasket before he ordered. On the evenings he headed directly home after work, Clark bought a hot pretzel while he waited for his train, if it was winter; in summer, he bought ice cream. When he finally walked into his house around 7 p.m., Clark devoured the leftovers from his kids' dinner or anything else he could get his hands on from the fridge while he waited to sit down with his wife for their dinner.

I once pointed out to Clark that during the day, he's so busy with his work that he can't stop to eat, and from 4 o'clock on, he can't stop eating.

After hearing similar stories of missed meals, grabbing food on the run, indiscriminate snacking and uncontrolled eating before and after dinner from others who *didn't* work on Wall Street, I realized that the Wall Street Eating Syndrome is actually a mirror of what is happening to society as a whole. We are shifting away from being a society that sits down to meals three times a day. Instead, people eat in motion. Most critically, breakfast and lunch are about grabbing whatever is quickest – or those meals are simply skipped entirely. Around 3 o'clock, just like the bell that rings on Wall Street to close the market, a hunger bell rings inside people and they start eating! Typically, people start grabbing whatever is around when their hunger gets too strong to ignore. They eat very quickly, so the food is not adequately digested and the body is never really satisfied by the meal. There are very few calories taken in during the early part of the day, and there is excessive calorie consumption from the late afternoon into the evening. Whenever a person is running short on time, time is 'borrowed' from breakfast or lunch. The quality of food is always secondary to how quickly it can be consumed. And a disproportionate amount of calories come from mindless nibbling on whatever food is around or from snack foods. There is little meal planning. There is even less *structure*.

WHAT IS STRUCTURE?

The structure of your eating habits is made up of these major components:

The timing and frequency of your meals

- Do you have established times to eat, and do you stick with them?
- Do you wait until you are hungry to eat?
- Do you skip any meals or replace them with snacks?
- Do you eat very quickly?

The type of meal you eat

- Is it a real meal or a quick snack in place of a meal?
- Is it adequate to carry you through the day?

How your home food shopping gets done

- What time of the day does it get done?
- What is bought?

The way your meals are served

- In serving dishes so everyone can help themselves?
- Individually plated?
- Do you eat meals standing up or while travelling?

Your eating structure is either a bridge to control or it promotes failure in weight loss. People with weight problems are most often people who have *no* structure at all in the critical areas of eating behaviour.

It's especially important that you begin by making sure that the timing, frequency and quality of your meals and snacks are structured to promote weight loss. This is what I mean:

- Eat breakfasts and lunches that contain sufficient protein and fibre, even if they must be quick meals that you eat while you multi-task.
- Eat a snack with both protein and fibre between 3 and 5 p.m.
- Don't go longer than 3 to 4 hours without a healthy meal or snack.
- Eat a dinner that contains a generous amount of high-fibre vegetables, a salad, and an adequate protein.
- *Never skip meals or snacks!*

The Worldwide Eating Syndrome?

Nutritionists have long puzzled over the so-called French Paradox or Italian Mystery because the French and Italian diets are rich in butters and cheeses, yet the French and Italians have less obesity-related disease than other Western countries, and in particular the US. What researchers have overlooked is that eating in France and Italy has long been *structured* into three meals a day, with an afternoon course of fruit or small cheese – with snacking being discouraged.

People in these countries do not skip meals (although Italians eat them later than many other Western countries). Random snacking is very rare. (Children are not given free rein with the refrigerator and microwave.) If you look into the pantry of an Italian or French kitchen, it is not loaded with junk food. Heavy desserts are reserved for holidays and special occasions. Many people in France and Italy still shop almost daily for fresh foods that they use completely in making one meal – as opposed to bringing enough food into the house each week to stock an air-raid shelter. It's neither a paradox nor a mystery: it's *structure!*

It is interesting to note that many of my European clients would consider it almost a form of child abuse to feed their children the sorts of junk food that many American clients are convinced their children can't live without. Perhaps that is the only paradox.

I have discovered that most of my weight clients skip either breakfast or lunch – and sometimes both – or eat inadequately at those meals. But almost no one ever skips dinner. Indeed, dinner is the meal where most people overconsume. Having seen the weight gains this lack of structure has caused in my clients, I am most concerned that you eat a proper breakfast and lunch so that you don't get too hungry as the day wears on and fall into the Wall Street Eating Syndrome.

The diet and menu section of this book has some specific suggestions for the ideal quick breakfast and lunch as well as delicious dinners. They may not take long to consume, but they will keep you satisfied and energetic. You will also find plenty of information about what constitutes a healthy snack.

NEVER LET A DIET MAKE YOU HUNGRY

The very biggest mistake any dieter can make is to skip meals or go too long without food. There is as much danger in eating too little when you are trying to lose weight as eating too much. If you let yourself become hungry, you will feel compelled to eat whatever you see first, and you will eat compulsively – or you'll be living with constant feelings of being deprived. Your own body has its own structure for eating, and unless the structure of your eating mirrors the body's structure, your weight can spin out of control.

Feeling hungry is not a sign that you are virtuously following your diet.

Feeling hungry is a sure sign that your diet is wrong or your eating habits are wrong.

We have a wealth of scientific studies that show that people who eat small nutritious meals frequently do much better with weight control than people who eat big meals infrequently. It's easy enough to see why: from your body's point of view, the very purpose of eating is to avoid hunger. If you do not feed your body adequate calories every 3 or 4 hours, then the next time you eat anything, you will set off a chemical chain reaction inside your body that makes you compulsively eat more.

What do I mean when I say 'adequate calories?' Your breakfast and lunch should be made up of foods that have enough nutrients to carry you through your busy day to the next meal without getting hungry. A small fat-free yogurt, for instance, is an excellent snack food, but it's not sufficient as a lunch by itself. If you look at the meal plans in this book, you will see that the structure of your meal should be built around providing your body with sufficient protein, fibre and other nutrients so that you are never hungry.

Some people tell me that when they are 'in the zone' to lose weight, it doesn't bother them to skip meals. But I have found that over a period of weeks, this skipping of meals invariably leads to cheating and losses of control with eating. Of all the thousands of people I've worked with, I can think of very few, if any, who skip meals on a regular basis and who kept their weight off. Perhaps that will convince you how important not skipping is.

Structure Is the Cravings Killer

There is another important reason why you should never go too long without eating. Almost all cravings come from what I call 'The Four S's': Seeing, Smelling, Stress and Starvation. In combination, the 'Four S's' throw a lethal curve at your ability to control what you eat. We are powerfully guided by our senses, which is a fact known to every modern advertiser and supermarket owner. They do everything they can to keep food in front of your eyes or get you to turn your head to look at it. And if they can get you to smell it when you're hungry, that's even better!

By giving yourself a solid structure of frequent meals and snacks every day, you protect yourself against the siren songs of the

Structure Right Now

One of the best ways to immediately structure your eating and shopping habits is to start keeping a food diary (see page 32), like the one I use with my own clients, which guides and reinforces structure. Studies on weight control indicate that people lose more weight when they keep a diary while on a weight programme.

Four S's. It's simply a physiological fact that if you go too long without eating, your blood sugar falls, and you are more prone to feel stressed and irritable. You may not be aware that you are setting yourself up to be overcome by cravings, since your mind is preoccupied with the activities of the day. But as soon as you encounter the sight or smell of a food that you like, it will have an impact on your appetite that is a thousand times more powerful than if you encountered those same foods on a full stomach. Your chances of being selective about what you eat and the amount you eat now are almost nonexistent!

As Dr C. Wayne Calloway, an endocrinologist at George Washington University, has observed, when you wait until you feel hungry before you eat, you jump-start the production of neuropeptide Y, which can lead to uncontrollable cravings, especially for carbohydrates. And once that happens, it's like losing the brake on your appetite, and you become 'an eating automaton'.

Dr Arthur Agatston, the famed author of *The South Beach Diet*, has warned that 'the carbohydrates that dominate the typical American diet – white bread, pasta, cereal, snack foods, cakes, cookies, candies, and so on – are stripped of fiber during processing. These foods are quickly digested and absorbed as glucose, the form sugar takes in the bloodstream. The body must produce increasing amounts of insulin to remove excess glucose in the blood.' Not only does this dangerously promote the storage of fat around the abdomen, Dr Agatston points out, 'high insulin levels end up removing too much glucose from the blood. The resulting low-blood sugar, called reactive hypoglycemia, triggers food cravings. The more you give in to your cravings, the more weight you gain.' Sadly, the overconsumption of these carbohydrates is no longer confined to the US, and is a major factor in rising obesity rates around the world.

If you go too long without eating and then you eat simple carbohydrates, you feel out of control with your appetite – you may even find yourself bingeing. This is a physiological phenomenon that many people incorrectly interpret as a psychological, emotional eating disorder. In truth, the disorder is completely physiological, caused by the lack of structure in your eating habits combined with the excessive consumption of simple carbohydrates.

ENDING FOOD CRAVINGS FOREVER

The best way to keep cravings from ruining your diet is to prevent them. Preventing anything in this world from happening, especially anything with a lot of history of occurring, requires planning and strategy. Prevention is preferable to rehabilitation, and it's much cheaper!

Planning and eating the right breakfast is the right strategy. Planning and eating the right lunch is the right strategy too. Both will keep you from having the feelings of hunger and dissatisfaction from cravings. Equally important: *eating a healthy snack every afternoon is an essential strategy in the prevention of food cravings, because it keeps your blood sugar stable and keeps hunger at bay.*

Still Balking at Eating Breakfast?

Some of my clients tell me that eating breakfast when they get up makes them more, not less, hungry as the morning wears on. Most of these clients were eating the wrong type of breakfast: one with too much sugar or too little fibre – or both. The biggest culprits seem to be sugary flaked cereals, bagels, croissants or even some kinds of oatmeal that are low in fibre (such as instant). If you have a history of becoming hungrier after eating breakfast, the first strategy to try is eating a *different kind of breakfast.* Experiment with the breakfast suggestions in the menu section of this book (see page 220), and focus on making a breakfast with protein. *Don't* skip breakfast altogether.

Some of my clients are simply never hungry when they get up. The answer for these people is to move their breakfast time to later in the morning, around 10.30 a.m. and then not eat lunch until 2 p.m. (The time of day is secondary, the structure of three meals and a snack sometime between lunch and dinner is primary.) Just make sure you always eat a breakfast. The universal laws of the human body require it.

The Cinderella Syndrome

Most of my clients suffer from what I call 'the Cinderella Syndrome'. For Cinderella, everything went south at midnight. For them, everything starts going south in the middle of the afternoon. Within a few hours after eating lunch, usually around 4 p.m., most people's blood sugar starts to dip. Unless they head off hunger with a truly healthy snack, as blood sugar goes lower and lower, people who are carbohydrate abusers tend to find themselves craving sweets or flour products. If you give in to that craving for simple carbohydrates, you trigger a chaotic cycle of chemical ups-and-downs that, by the time dinnertime rolls around, will make you a compulsive eater instead of a selective one. If you find this craving cycle is a factor in your life, you can end it with two simple steps:

1. Remind yourself (if you're craving sweets or junk snacks): this is not about sweets or junk. It's 4 p.m., and my blood sugar is low. That's why I want something sweet.

2. Eat a low-fat protein snack such as a fat-free/low-fat yogurt with some fresh berries, or another low-sugar fruit or a protein with fibre such as my recommended low-fat cheese with the high-fibre bran crackers (such as Laughing Cow Light Cheese Triangles with GG Scandinavian Bran Crispbread). Other people find that an apple with one of the cheese triangles or a protein shake works brilliantly. (The protein shake should be no more than 100 calories per serving. Few ready-made ones are that low so you may need to buy a protein powder from a health food shop and mix your own.)

YOUR THINPACK: NEVER LEAVE HOME WITHOUT IT!

Life is unpredictable. I teach my clients never to be without an extra healthy snack in their bag or briefcase. That's so they will never have to worry that they might lose to a snack bar or a bag of peanuts when life throws them an unexpected crisis, and their next meal is delayed. Having a smart food strategy means that you, too, will never succumb to eating the biscuits at a conference or school event for your kids and that you will never grab fattening food on the run. It also means you will *never* be hungry.

Since we live in a very busy world, I've come up with a perfect way to guarantee that you'll never be battling cravings because you've gone too long without eating: a ThinPack!

What's a ThinPack?

It's a self-sealing bag that contains two or three high-fibre crackers (such as the GG Scandinavian Bran Crispbread), an apple and two low-fat, pre-wrapped cheese wedges (such as Mini-Babybel Lights or Laughing Cow Light), which can go for a few hours without refrigeration. If cheese is a trigger food for you, substitute slices of low-fat cold meat or 2 tablespoons of peanut butter for a delicious sandwich with the crackers, or any other form of protein *that you have no history of abusing*. Beware of shelled nuts as these are tricky for some – light popcorn in a small bag provides a delicious, high-fibre substitute.

With your ThinPack right at hand at all times, you can weather any delay or unexpected change in your schedule.

Dinner after 7?

Many of my clients get into trouble because their partner gets home from work later than they do, and they become ravenously hungry waiting to eat dinner. Some end up eating their kids' food while they wait, others keep picking at the dinner ingredients, eating bread and snack foods, or they just don't eat anything and gorge at dinner.

If you aren't likely to have dinner within 4 hours of your afternoon snack, add an early evening snack to your daily menu plan, preferably one with protein and fibre, such as a small serving of cheese with an apple or bran crackers, or a tomato juice and celery with virtually fat-free cream cheese (look for Quark or Weight Watchers soft cheese). Or, for about the same number of calories, have a mini-meal such as an egg-white omelette with vegetables, or a couple of scoops of my Dilled Egg Salad (see page 237).

We were wrongly told as children 'Don't spoil your dinner!' when we reached for a snack while waiting for the adults to make supper. Since most weight clients consume the greatest amount of their calories around dinnertime, get rid of that outdated advice. Never go hungry to dinner. Don't worry about spoiling your appetite; worry about spoiling your figure or your weight loss!

THIN STARTS IN THE SUPERMARKET

I tell my clients that they should never walk into any type of super-market, farmer's market or speciality food store if they are hungry. (Eat first, and wait for the hunger to pass.) And never go shopping without a list. Wandering around a supermarket looking for things to buy almost guarantees that you will automatically buy many of the same foods that made you fat. Also, it only stimulates your curiosity to try new foods – on top of what already is tempting you. If you have a problem with snack foods or junk foods, it's not a good idea to go shopping with your children, because the pack-aging on many unhealthy foods is designed to attract a child's interest. You'll likely end up with a kitchen full of snack foods that will undermine your weight-loss programme.

I also strongly discourage my clients from doing *any* food shopping after work. Most people are mentally fatigued and hungry at the end of the day, which means they're more likely to succumb to impulse buying when they are surrounded by the sights and smells of food. By contrast, very few people feel any urge to overeat in the morning.

The best time to go food shopping is right after breakfast or right after eating. The worst time is between 3 and 6 p.m. If you must shop at this time, eat a healthy snack first.

With a satisfied stomach, you'll be less tempted by the brightly coloured, alluring packaging of junk foods and frozen desserts and the aromas of fresh baked goods.

My client Eva switched to doing her shopping on Sunday mornings after breakfast, and not only did she find the supermarket less crowded than during the evening 'rush hour', she more easily lost weight than she had before. Dorothy, who is a single mother, tried switching to shopping on Saturday mornings instead of doing it on her way home from work, but she discovered that her kids would want to go with her and then it was much harder to control what went into the shopping trolley. Dorothy went back to shop-ping after work, but on her way to the supermarket, she drinks a small can of V-8 juice and eats a sandwich made of bran crackers and low-fat cold meat. Her shopping hours no longer interfere with her weight loss. Pick the strategy that works best for your weight loss. Just make sure you *never* enter a food store feeling hungry.

MEAL STRUCTURE AND THE 'E.A.T. PRINCIPLE'

Your meals and snacks themselves can and should have a firm structure that optimizes your control over eating. Buffets and all-you-can-eat restaurants offer only *unstructured* eating. So does dining 'family style' at home (where everybody serves themselves from large dishes that are passed around the table). Snacking directly from a supersize bag of potato crisps or picking over an entire bunch of grapes on the kitchen counter is also eating without structure. Eating foods and meals without structure is a prelude to excessive consumption and losses of control.

Shopping with Structure

Before you take your next trip to the supermarket, review these tips, and keep them in mind as you're walking up and down the aisles.

Beware the 'bargain size'! People who buy bargain-size bags of food get no bargain at all. They end up spending the few pennies they save on larger-size clothing and, far worse, prescription medications.

Buy your food in structures that help you eat less. Buy as much of your food as you can packaged in units that minimize the possibility of your over-consuming or having any leftovers from your meal or your snack. People always eat less when presented with individual-ized servings and tend to eat much more from large bags and boxes – remember people are finishers.

Stick to your list. Always make a shopping list before you enter the supermarket, even if you have to stand outside the door and write one up. Inside the shop, *stick to your list!* You don't need a food just because it's on sale. Yes, over time, you wind up paying a little more at the checkout each week when you live inside a good structure, but you get a priceless payoff in good health and a happier life.

Don't buy foods for others that you have a history of abusing, unless they specifically ask for them. If they do, buy the smallest size possible, and ask them to keep it out of your sight. If you do buy snack foods for others, buy ones that are not your favourites to reduce temptation.

Through my work with thousands of weight clients, I have discovered what I consider to be something close to a law of human nature. I call it 'E.A.T.' or the Expanding Appetite Theorem: *appetite expands to consume the amount of food presented.* If you are served 4 ounces of food, you will eat 4 ounces of food. If you are served 8 ounces, you will eat 8 ounces. If you go to buffet-style restaurants, you will eat more than if you go to a restaurant where all your food is put on a plate for you alone by the chef. If you buy the largest bag of popcorn at the movies, you will eat far more popcorn than if you buy the smallest.

But I've also discovered that there is an equal force in nature that opposes E.A.T.: *the more precisely structured your food is, the less likely you are to overeat it.* An example? You will always eat only one serving of potato if it's baked, but you may not know when to stop if it's mashed. Similarly, people will often eat far fewer calories in a restaurant if they order a baked potato with their main course instead of rice. One restaurant serving of rice can be anything from a few tablespoons to half a plateful, and most people will finish all that is served to them. The larger portion does not give any greater sense of satiety of satisfaction than the smaller one does. We simply eat the extra amount just because it's there.

The same applies to fresh fruits you eat for a dessert or snack. Have you ever eaten more than one apple at a time? But you're

Have You Got Unophobia?

I've noticed that hundreds, perhaps even thousands, of my clients feel deprived and depressed if they see one lonely piece of anything on their plate, whether it is one slice of bread or an egg. But they instantly cheer up if their food has a mate. If you're 'unophobic', cut your serving into two pieces! It's amazing how much more satisfied people feel eating two halves of a peach instead of a whole one or one hard-boiled egg that's been sliced into quarters. Similarly, you'll be much more satisfied with two pieces of 40-calorie light wheat bread than with one piece of the regular wheat bread for 80 calories.

likely to eat too many cherries or pineapple chunks if you dish them out of a big bowl or tin. In the summer, many of my clients have seen their weight loss stop or diminish because they keep bowls of cut-up fruit in the refrigerator and overeat it constantly.

People eat with their eyes as much as they eat with their mouths. The larger the serving or the availability, the more you will eat. I strongly advise my clients to run away from the food 'minis': mini-muffins, mini-doughnuts, mini-cookies, and even mini-fruits such as prunes or mandarin oranges.

It seems that many of my male clients don't realize that, at social events, they eat far more calories during the cocktail hour picking at bite-size finger foods than they eat during the entire dinner itself. The food 'minis' either fool you into believing you're barely eating at all or that you can't be eating too many calories, since the serving size is so small. And they make it too easy for you to lose count of how much you're eating.

If you eat like the intelligent people who sit in my office, you'll consume more calories eating the 'minis' than you would have had you simply served yourself one normal portion of food. (The only exception I make to my 'anti-mini' rule is low-fat mini-cheeses that are individually sealed in wax or foil. Dieters are less likely to overeat these premeasured servings that have to be unwrapped than if they try to slice a small portion of cheese from a block. The cheese block becomes like the bowl of cut-up fruit. People keep going back for instant, repeat servings.)

STRUCTURE EMPOWERS YOU TO DO THE RIGHT THING

Structure prevents the cravings and hunger that tempt you to violate your diet. It guides you in planning your meals and snacks and your food shopping. It guides you to being protective of yourself and honouring your body's needs. *When people structure their eating habits, within a week or two they feel back in control of their life again.* By eating at regular intervals, your *hunger* has dissipated and your cravings have dissipated, even though you are eating a fraction of the calories you were eating before.

You no longer feel like a failure, and why should you ever?

Strategies for Buffets, All-You-Can-Eat Restaurants and Cocktail Parties

Here are some hints and tips to put into action when you know you're going to be faced with a lot of food in a social setting.

Eat a snack before you go out to eat or to a party.

Say to yourself before you walk in: 'I've seen it all and tasted it all before; there's nothing really new. It's glorified cafeteria food.'

Put Listerine Breath Strips on your tongue before you enter to block the tempting aromas.

Drink a glass of tomato juice or a Virgin Bloody Mary when you arrive.

Do not survey the entire buffet.

Pick the smallest plate or a child's plate to serve yourself, not an oversize dinner plate.

Say to yourself before you put any food on your plate: 'If I eat it all, I will wear it all.'

Take only one main course dish or two half servings. Then go directly to the vegetable and salad section. Avoid vegetables or salads sitting in oil or butter.

Strive to make your plate look like a regular restaurant plate of food.

Don't survey the dessert section if desserts are your issue.

Say to yourself after you've eaten one serving: 'It's more important to get my life's worth than my money's worth.'

At a cocktail party or standing buffet, carry a clutch bag plus a beverage, or a cup and saucer. If your hands are full, you can't eat.

Structure is not only part of a successful *diet*. It must remain part of a successful eating style. The reason so many people succeed at weight loss but fail at weight maintenance is that once their clothes fit better, they get loose with structure. And once they are loose about structure, they fall back into the throes of old cravings and temptations. This is a certainty, so if you want lasting success, remember: *structure gives control – and structure guards control.*

Happy or sad, rich or poor…it's still better being thin.
Even if you want to be miserable today, it's better to be
thin and miserable than fat and miserable.

The Fifth Thin Commandment:

Separate Mood from Food

COMMANDMENT ESSENTIALS

- Don't buy snacks you habitually abuse when you are stressed.
- Keep tempting snack foods (that you must have on hand for family members) out of sight.
- Keep healthy snack foods available.
- Pick up the phone and chat with a friend instead of picking up a potato crisp or biscuit.
- Practise yoga, weed your garden, knit or do some other activity instead of stress eating.
- Switch to a stress food substitute that won't make you fat.
- Talk yourself out of mood eating.

SOMETIMES EATING IS NOT about food.

Emotional eating is one of the most pervasive and over-whelming issues for dieters to deal with. It's also one of the most insidious, because no matter how much weight you lose, if the next time you get upset, you return to your old ways, your castle is built on sand.

Diets that focus on caloric thinking have no answers for people who have a history of mood eating. They offer no strategies to

block it or end it. As long as we approach dieting with an oversim-
plified model of calories in and calories out, the very high failure
rate for dieters will remain what it is because we have lost sight of
the human being who is the most important factor in the equation.
In dealing with a human behaviour, one plus one often does not
equal two. There is logic – and there is *psycho*logic.

At the opposite extreme, unfortunately, most discussions of
mood eating are overloaded with psychobabble. Since I have a background in a branch of psychology that explores human motivation
rather than psychopathology, I didn't enter the field of weight control with a belief that just because a person has gained weight, he
must have some hidden psychological problem. As I have said
before, *we don't have to be crazy to be crazy about a cookie!*

The obvious reason that people use a food to change their
mood is that the food they are abusing *tastes* good. Almost all mood
eaters reach for snacks with a sweet taste or creamy texture, or they
want a crunchy texture that is salty or sweet. Those tastes and textures provide mood eaters with *immediate satisfaction*. Crunching on
something may actually relieve pent-up emotions in the same way
pummelling a pillow would. And when you keep lots of such snack
foods around your house, eating to change your emotions becomes
more user-friendly and immediate.

I will never tell you that the foods you choose to eat as mood
lifters don't have a pleasurable taste. They do. But nothing tastes
better than looking in the mirror every morning and feeling proud
of what you see. Food pleasure is fleeting, and I've yet to meet the
stress eater who is happy with his behaviour or himself for doing it!

Mood eating is a learned behaviour, and fortunately, whatever
has been learned can be unlearned, even if we learned it long ago
and have strengthened the lessons through habit. The good news is
that even though mood eating is one of the most pervasive and
insidious challenges faced by dieters and traditional weight-control
programmes, it is one of the most amenable to correct through
strategy. When you look closely at actual histories of mood eaters,
you make a liberating discovery.

*For the overwhelming majority, mood eating isn't about food – and it's
not about fine dining. It's about snacking and grabbing whatever is around
in your immediate environment that looks 'interesting'.*

My client Sonia loves to cook, but when she gets stressed, she doesn't drop everything to bake her favourite lasagne. She'll just raid her kids' cookie jar. Craig truly enjoys gourmet food, but when he has a lousy day at the office, he doesn't slip into a fine restaurant and order three main courses. He'll eat a large-size bag of crisps on his way home. Marilyn's New York apartment is right down the street from an all-night gourmet food store, but every time she gets an aggravating phone call from her sister, she'll only binge on ice cream as long as she doesn't have to walk one step further than the fridge to get it!

So the pattern is clear: mood eating isn't about food. It's about snacking and grabbing whatever is around. *Mood eating is about immediacy – right now.*

What mood eaters want is an *immediate* change in their feelings. That's why it's about *snacking* not real food, and it's about snacking on what's easiest to get into your mouth. In all the years I've been working on weight control in the most stress-ridden city in America, the number of clients I've had who reacted to stress by cooking, shopping or dining in restaurants is so small that, while I can't say I can count the number on the fingers of two hands, I don't need many more fingers than that. I've worked successfully with thousands of stress eaters, and despite their sex differences, and diverse backgrounds, and economic status, I would estimate that close to 90 per cent shared this single common pattern when it came to mood eating:

- **Same food.** Mood eaters return time and time again to their favourite snack food – a snack that is either crunchy (such as potato crisps, crackers, pretzels or even cereal); sweet (such as biscuits and confectionery); or creamy (such as ice cream or frozen yogurt). Most typically, they prefer a bite-size food that they can keep popping into their mouths, almost independent of whether they are hungry or not.

- **Same place.** Mood eaters eat alone in the kitchen. A very small number do their mood eating at their office.

- **Same time of day.** Mood eating is done in the late afternoon or evening, almost never in the morning.

- **Same moods.** It's feelings of anxiety, anger, frustration, betrayal, disappointment or boredom that are the common triggers for mood eating.

- **Same people.** Mood eaters snack because they become stressed by the same *people* over and over again (such as a boss, a partner, a child, a relative or a friend).
- **Same situations.** Mood eaters snack because they become stressed by the same *situations* over and over again (such as having to make presentations at work or being in uncomfortable social situations), or they're bored, and eating becomes 'something interesting to do'.
- **Same quantities of food.** Mood eating is almost always about volume. Whether one is dealing with frustration or boredom, a mood doesn't evaporate with one M&M. As the mood lingers, people want the eating to linger also, so they choose snacks with a 'long-eating' time – like a bag of M&Ms.
- **Same reason.** Mood eaters want a treat or comfort from the food. That is why mood eating is almost always done with a food they buy and bring home for themselves, even if they may believe they bought it for others, especially their family or company.

Are You a Boredom Eater?

One of the surprising things I've discovered about boredom eaters is that, unlike other mood eaters, the act of snacking is more important to them than what they snack on. While most mood eaters aren't really happy unless they can munch their favourite snacks, boredom eaters will eat anything so long as it fills up time, and they can easily pick at it from the kitchen counter, the refrigerator or cupboard.

Planning is the cure for boredom eating. Designing a flower bed, reading an interesting book, sending e-mails to your friends or just about any activity you can think of that's legal is a better use of your time than boredom eating!

But even the most organized people can end up with unstructured time on their hands. If you are a boredom eater, keep a plate of raw vegetables in your refrigerator or a single bag of light popcorn you can chew on. Especially avoid bringing home the fascinating 'finger food' you see in the shops, like nuts and flavoured crackers, and never use food shopping as an escape from tedium. When simple boredom turns into high-fat boredom eating, people can end up literally bored to death.

If you're a frequent mood eater, there's a very good chance that you do it because of the same moods caused by the same people and same situations that caused you stress before, and you do your mood eating alone in the same place, at the same time of day, and with the same food nearly every time.

Once you realize your mood eating is totally predictable, you can control it with strategy!

Judy was an extremely intelligent hospital executive who came to me after a number of therapists failed to help her control her mood eating. 'Why do I keep doing this,' she asked angrily in my office, 'when I know I'm just eating out of stress and tension? I'm not even hungry!' As I asked her questions about her eating patterns, it became clear that Judy always made a beeline for any kind of sweet, baked food that was also a finger food, such as cookies. She never went for the snacks her husband had around the house, because she didn't like his salty, crunchy foods.

I couldn't help but ask Judy, 'Why do you keep buying *your* type of snack food and bringing it home when you know you're a mood eater?'

THE BEST PLACE TO END MOOD EATING FOREVER

The best place to end mood eating is not a psychiatrist's couch. It's the supermarket. If you know you have a tendency to eat when you are upset, don't buy the snacks you habitually abuse when you are stressed or bring them into the house because your own kitchen is probably where you do most of your mood eating.

The interesting and even wonderful thing about ending the pattern of mood eating is that when snacks aren't immediately available, almost all mood eaters automatically busy themselves with a *noneating* activity, such as watching TV, listening to music or cleaning, which disperses their energy. In the end, no matter what the burdens and stresses of your life may be, you can't eat what's not there! But mood eaters can't get beyond compulsive snacking if they keep their kitchen stocked with convenient snacks.

Once Judy stopped stocking up with all her favourite snack foods, she was astonished that her mood eating disappeared, and her subsequent weight loss was significant. 'I never dreamed I could do it so easily,' she marvelled 2 months later, by which time she was already one dress size smaller. Judy had become even more fit by putting a Ping-Pong table in her basement to work out her stresses with her kids.

Buying or having your favourite snack foods in the house encourages and reinforces the destructive habit of mood eating. I've learned that quite a few of my clients are like Peter, who works from home as a computer consultant. It used to be that whenever Peter had peanut M&Ms in his house, he magnified every minor setback that came along during the day into an excuse to eat. When his Internet connection went down, when a delivery didn't arrive, Peter decided he 'needed' a snack break. Peter does most of the family shopping, and he insisted that the only reason he bought the family-size bags of peanut M&Ms was because his kids ate them too. But his kids almost never saw any of them! Peter switched to buying fruit sweets for his kids and stopped bringing peanut M&Ms into the house, and his own 'stress' snacking stopped. He not only lost his spare tyre, Peter claims he has the best-organized home office in town!

Strategies for Snack Foods

If you know your favourite nibble is right in the next room, the least provocation or annoyance can become the excuse to indulge. The very availability of the snack creates conscious and unconscious rationalizations to keep on eating it.

Why not employ a strategy right now, and toss out the 'mood snacks' that are in your kitchen? When you make up your next shopping list, simply don't add those foods to your list – and while you are in the supermarket, please stick to your list. If someone else does the family shopping, ask for their cooperation in making you slim.

If you absolutely must keep snacks in your home for other people, here are proven strategies to keep you from eating them:

• Ask others in your home for permission to buy a type of snack that is not your favourite or that you are unlikely to abuse. If they insist on having a snack that tempts you, buy only a single serving for them, and give it to them immediately to keep. (It's always a smart strategy to buy *all* snacks in single, individually wrapped servings, because snacks are a type of food that is so easy to overconsume.)

• Keep snack foods out of sight. Take all snack foods out of their highly attractive packaging, and keep them in plain brown bags or containers that aren't transparent. Another good strategy is to keep snacks behind a cupboard door that you rarely open or that is out of your line of vision, or keep them at the back of your most hard-to-reach shelf. *Never keep snacks on the kitchen worktop or table.* It encourages mindless snacking. The kitchen worktop is the single most dangerous spot in your house for your weight-control efforts. It's easily accessible, and it's the first thing people see and reach for (whether they are hungry or not) when there is food on it.

• Ask those in your immediate family and your good friends not to snack in front of you whenever possible.

• Have family members hide tempting snack foods if you're given to grazing.

• If nothing else works, lock all snacks in a cash box with a combination lock, and make sure only those who eat the snacks enclosed have the combination.

• Keep healthy snack foods available (like an apple or cut-up vegetables), so you're not tempted to go for any fattening ones that are around.

Remember: living your life trim and healthy is far more important than spending extra money on a lockbox or worrying that a strategy looks 'crazy'. The only thing that's crazy is your looking fat because you're going down the tubes again and again for snack food!

When we dispense with the need to be normal, life gets so much easier! I am convinced that one of the reasons my clients are so successful at losing weight and keeping it off is that they are able to think outside the box. They quickly learn not to ask: 'Is this normal?' They just respect what works. What works for you *is* what's normal for your life!

IS IT REALLY A CRISIS?

Carl was a longtime client of mine whose beloved father had a stroke. Carl spent entire days and nights at the hospital, and I only learned of the situation when Carl's wife called me to say that she was alarmed because Carl had eaten very little for days. Despite his long history of mood eating, Carl is like most of us: when we are profoundly upset, we lose our appetite.

It's actually the *day-to-day annoyances*, not the profound upsets, that prompt mood eaters to reach for their snacks. Almost all mood eating is really about simply getting rid of a stressful day or event. It's about immediately substituting a pleasurable feeling for an unpleasant one. That's why when the shock of a genuine crisis hits us, it never occurs to us to open up a bag of crisps.

The key to controlling mood eating is recognizing that the vast majority of the time, the kind of stress that does make us want to eat is *predictable* stress: it is stress that comes from the same familiar people and the same familiar situations time and time again.

Strategies for Stress on the Horizon

If your youngest child is starting kindergarten next week; if your older brother spoils every family occasion and your parents' 40th anniversary is coming up; if you'll have to deliver last quarter's disappointing sales report to management on Thursday, you have every reason in the world to plan in advance what you are going to eat on those days. One day of stress really doesn't have to become a legacy of fat.

When stress looms, I have found that three simple techniques dramatically reduce the likelihood of your turning to food to relieve the stress:

Write out what you will eat for that day in advance. Create a sample menu for what you will eat for breakfast, lunch, dinner and snacks. Direct your psyche to think in terms of these foods only and to avoid all others.

Plan which snacks you are going to eat, and keep all others out of sight. (When making up your ThinPack, you probably want the items for a predictable 'stress day' to have some crunch.)

Plan to avoid trouble. Don't drive down a road that takes you past your favourite bakery on a day when you know you'll be stressed out. Take all the change out of your pockets before you walk to the conference room if you know you'll have to pass the vending machines.

I've almost always found that when people plan what they're going to eat on a 'stress day' and how they're going to stay away from trouble, they're able to get through any stressful situation successfully.

Give Your Stress a Dress Rehearsal

Many mood-eating clients find it very helpful to mentally rehearse what they expect to encounter from a stressful person or situation. If it's a person who is surely going to give you trouble, you can tell yourself: 'I know what she is going to say and how she's going to react.' You can rehearse the words you fear hearing in your own mind until they lose their power to provoke you. Also rehearse what you will say or do in response. Mentally walking yourself through a dreaded situation several times in advance can dispel a lot of anxiety and make you feel confident of your ability to control the situation, including your eating.

A WINNER ALWAYS PLANS FOR THE UNKNOWN

We all know not every stressful day is predictable. Life happens! It throws up unexpected events. Even when you already know that it's mainly your kids or colleagues who cause you to feel stressed, you can't always predict *when* a day that begins as a breeze will snowball into disaster. Your kids don't plan to break expensive lamps. Your colleagues don't plan to make the computer system crash. The winners at weight control don't let the unknown catch them unprepared.

'Planning is stronger than willpower!' is the motto that all my former mood eaters live by. They've come to appreciate the beauty of planning in keeping stress from turning into fat!

You can join them in the winner's circle of weight control by making their winning strategies your own. If you haven't done it already, make a list of your friends' telephone numbers, so you can dial them easily when stress next hits. Decide right now that the next time you feel a bad mood rising, you'll spend a few minutes doing a favourite activity, especially one that occupies your hands. (Ex-smokers in particular should look for ways to keep their hands busy, so they don't start picking at fattening finger foods.)

My client Daniel throws darts at a wooden bull's-eye that he hung on the back of his office door. Alice's ongoing project is to arrange her CD collection into perfect order. (You can listen to music while you do it!) Laura sorts through her holiday photos and puts them into albums. If you have a drawer at home or in your office that's become a dumping ground, you might promise yourself that the next time you're upset, you'll straighten out that drawer.

A reader of *More* magazine recently wrote to its editors to say: 'When I pick up my knitting, I feel an instantaneous physical response. My blood pressure drops and I experience a calmness throughout my body. Knitting is my yoga!'

If you're a mood eater, it's wise to find *your* yoga! (Maybe yoga *is* your yoga!) If you don't have a healthy, constructive outlet for stress, look for one you'd like to adopt. Focus on activities that you can do at home that don't require an elaborate setup, so you'll be able to turn to them immediately. Try to avoid activities that are so demanding that they might frustrate you or increase your stress. And make sure the activity you choose interests you enough that boredom doesn't tempt you to eat!

Best Activities to Block Stress Eating

Don't let stress get the better of you and your weight. The next time you feel stressed out, try one of these activities instead of heading for the kitchen.

Knitting and crocheting
Taking a warm bath or shower
Playing with a Game Boy
Playing with a pet
Reciting a favourite poem or prayer
Keeping a diary
Sending e-mails to friends

Going online to learn about
  something that interests you
Having sex
Stretching and exercising, especially
  with hand weights
Meditation or yoga
Squeezing a rubber ball
Watching a video or reading a
  compelling book
Playing an instrument
Shopping for items you enjoy (other
  than food)

IF YOU CAN'T STOP IT, SWITCH IT

In a perfect world, I would tell you that the best way to rid yourself of your stress is to always stop what you are doing, exercise vigorously, or take a warm bath. Science suggests this is the best route, but sometimes – in fact, most times – life doesn't give us this opportunity.

My client Nancy is a mood eater who told me before I'd even offered her a list of strategies that she didn't have the time or energy for diversions when she's stressed out. Nancy has toddler twins and a 5-year-old who keep her running in three different directions every minute of the day. By the time she manages to get them all to sleep each night, the only thing Nancy can think about doing is curling up in an easy chair with a magazine and a packet of biscuits. She'd keep eating biscuits as she read, and she'd end up eating as many as a dozen.

We all have to work with the way our lives really are, not the way other people tell us they should be. My job is to help my clients stay trim without asking them to enter monasteries or submit to personality transplants. *One of my great surprises was to learn that most stress eaters are very open to switching to foods that have similar characteristics to the foods they abuse, but which aren't fattening. They will even feel better immediately if they switch to a food that is healthy for them.*

Typically, people are looking for just two things from their 'stress' snack: they want it immediately at hand, and they want it to be pleasurable. So I suggested to Nancy that instead of snacking on biscuits, she switch to wholegrain waffles and a diet hot chocolate. The next time I saw her, Nancy told me she was delighted with the switch: the crunchy waffle was easy to make and delicious. Because of its high-fibre content, a wholegrain waffle gave her enough of a feeling of satisfaction that it replaced all 12 biscuits she had been eating. Nancy told me that the diet hot chocolate, which was only 35 calories, added an extra dimension of relaxation to the end of her day.

Crunch a Bunch of Healthy Snacks

Jack is a statistician who spends long hours in front of his computer, building up tensions that have no place to go. By the time he gets home, Jack is too tired to go to sleep or do much except watch TV.

Stress Substitutes That Won't Make You Fat

If you absolutely have to reach for a snack when stressed, it doesn't have to be something that's going to add on the pounds. Here's a quick glance at the foods that spell trouble in times of stress – and healthy substitutes that won't sabotage your diet.

The Dangers

Biscuits and cookies, especially small ones

Chocolates

Chewy confectionery such as gummy bears

Crunchy *thin* crackers that are salty and flavourful

Crunchy or sweetened cereals

Potato crisps

Pretzels

Mounds of cheese you can keep picking on

Nuts and savoury snack mixes

Finger fruits such as grapes, cherries and raisins

Hors d'oeuvres

The Healthy Substitutes

Bran crackers with or without fat-free soft cheese (Quark)

Rice cakes

Fruit ice pops

Sugar-free gum, preferably one that's not sweet (try Dentyne)

A chilled beverage, such as sugar-free lemonade or flavoured mineral water

A creamy low-calorie beverage (for an ice cream substitute), such as a protein shake or hot chocolate

Light popcorn *only* in individual serving bags

Crispbreads, such as GG Scandinavian brand

Thin soups in individual servings (instant)

Sunflower seeds in *individual* snack bags

Raw green vegetables, such as peppers, celery and fennel

Individual-size low-fat cheeses that have to be unwrapped before you can eat them, such as Laughing Cow Lights

But Jack has never been able to sit in front of the tube without crunching on something. By the time he walked into my office, he weighed more than 136 kg (300 lb).

Jack wasn't particular about what he crunched. When I suggested to Jack that he toss out the junk snacks and substitute as many raw green beans as he wanted to eat, Jack's eyes lit up. As a health statistician, Jack knew full well that green beans are loaded with disease-fighting phytonutrients. Jack made the switch that night, and like many of my clients, he's now sailing along as a trim person snacking on raw vegetables.

Smart food strategy has the power to shift dangerous behaviour in the direction of benign behaviour. It liberated Jack and my other clients from the destructive cycle of 'stress, eat, get fat'. Smart food strategy removed the most painful part of the cycle: the negative consequence. Jack still crunches nonstop on green beans while he watches TV, but the consequence now is a positive one.

By overconsuming non-fattening vegetables instead of junk food, you're actually extending your life and reducing the risk factors for many serious diseases. Just making the switch from junk food to a health-giving food will give you a feeling of greater power over your life.

WHY WEIGHT LOSS IS BETTER THAN PROZAC

When it comes to mood elevation, I have found that all the chocolates of Belgium, all the pizza of Italy, or all the ice cream of Häagen-Dazs will never elevate mood as much as losing weight, looking better and feeling in control again. The most effective Prozac in the world is to take charge of your weight. I have a favourite mantra: 'Happy or sad, rich or poor, it's still better being thin!' Even if you want to be miserable today, it's better to be thin and miserable than fat and miserable. Anyway you look at it, thin comes out ahead!

If eating could make people happy, then the heaviest people in the world would be the happiest. We all know that's not true, yet it's very easy to understand why we so often lose sight of it: there is massive confusion in our society between pleasure and happiness. The heroin user, shooting that drug into her vein, has such feelings of pleasure that it overcomes the normal human revulsion to pain and needles. But that very pleasure destroys the possibility of happiness in a human life.

When you think about all the pain caused by the gaining and regaining of weight as a result of mood eating, you realize that 'comfort foods' are a major cause of *discomfort* in human life. It's important that we realize that there are destructive pleasures – and that what we learned to be a benign comfort of our childhood may have become a destructive pleasure of our adulthood.

One of the most destructive aspects of mood eating goes almost totally unrecognized – mood eating deceives us into living as mimics. When someone hurts or disappoints you, you then disappoint yourself by breaking with your weight programme and gaining weight simply because you were eating as a result of *their* behaviour. It's rather ironic that when we eat because someone or something has made us angry or upset, we then also get angry with ourselves for doing it. It's a no-win pattern.

If you stop and reflect, most of the annoyances that prompt you to mood-eat – whether it's children's behaviour or a comment made by a boss or relative – are not as important as the harm you do to your body and psyche by perpetuating a cycle of mood eating. By perpetuating this cycle, you perpetuate a sense of being unable to cope without dependence on food.

Many of my clients who faced terrible crises during the time they were working with me have told me that applying these new strategies that prevented them from turning to chocolates or peanuts became one of the greatest sources of strength in their lives. Whenever you use strategy, it puts you in control. Strategy empowers you to deal with the agenda of your life. You are no longer reacting as a victim but are the leader in your own life.

Your lifelong success at weight control depends on how well you handle the foods that tempt you the most.

The Sixth Thin Commandment:
Take Control of
Your Favourite Foods

COMMANDMENT ESSENTIALS

- Limit frequency, availability and quantity of your favourite foods.
- Make 'I don't begin; I don't have any problem' your mantra and use it.
- Save your calories for special meals, not everyday junk.
- Remember to think historically.
- Don't request the dessert menu 'just for a look'.

LET'S FACE IT: many of your favourite foods are high in calories, and some of them may have got you into trouble in the past. But that doesn't mean you can't still enjoy them.

With a smart game plan, you can eat your favourite foods without having to wear them.

As so many of the winners at weight control have discovered, the dual strategies of *Box It In* and *Box It Out* are powerful solutions that make it easy to succeed at keeping high-calorie foods in your life without gaining weight. You don't have to give up the treats you love. *These techniques let you take control of your favourite foods, so they don't take control of you.*

To *Box In* a food means you include it in your diet. The goal is always to keep as many favourite foods as possible in your life – and also to keep wearing your favourite size.

To *Box Out* means you exclude a food or type of food (such as bite-size snacks that are easy to pop into your mouth) from your diet. For some people, certain foods create such powerful cravings that they need to be treated separately. And although that may sound difficult, the majority of my clients have told me that among all the skills they've developed for managing their weight, Box It Out is the single most effective, easy-to-use way to maintain success at weight control.

Together, Box It In and Box It Out provide a set of tools that can free you forever from overeating your problem foods – and still let you enjoy them without gaining weight.

BOXING IN YOUR FAVOURITE FOODS

Eating much-loved foods without putting on pounds is exactly what trips up so many people in their weight-control efforts. It may be the biggest stumbling block that you have faced over and over in the past. So, obviously, *this is one of the central issues of weight-control success.*

To stay trim and still eat what you love is a real skill – and an important mark of the winners at weight control. *The strategy that will allow you to master your favourite foods, once and for all, may be the most powerful tool you can take from this book.* For thousands of my clients, it's brought a permanent victory over their weight by controlling calories, limiting temptations and ending their continual struggle with food.

Let's start by looking at the techniques that can help you to be thin for life, too.

1. **Limit frequency.** Enjoy your favourite food only at a specified time. Have it on designated days, or only in certain restaurants, or when served to you at a party. Whether you include it in your diet regularly or only on special occasions will depend on the food and your personal history with it.

2. **Limit availability.** Keep tempting foods out of your line of vision at home, and avoid eye contact with them in restaurants and at other social events. One of the major triggers for

wanting something is seeing it and smelling it. The studies on eating behaviour are very clear about a simple fact: the more you see and are around the fattening foods you love, the more you will be tempted to eat them, the more you'll have cravings to battle and the more you'll weigh. Being in control at home makes it easier to be in charge outside. If you're sloppy with your food consumption in private, it will have a ripple effect in public.

3. **Limit quantity.** Buy your favourite food in single serving sizes, serve it only in individual portions and don't store it in large quantities.

Paula, a pediatrician with a fondness for desserts, allows herself to eat pies and cakes, but she lives by the rule that she will never buy a dessert for herself and take it home. She can order it out or enjoy it when it's offered to her at the home of a friend, although she holds herself to no more than once a week.

She also allows herself to bake a sweet course when she's entertaining, but she prepares the dessert in individual portions so there are no extras to tempt her. If any is left over, she sends it home with someone else or quietly throws it out *before* the last guest leaves. Paula knows that by establishing how often she eats the food that she finds the most seductive and by reducing her opportunity to be around it, she can stay on track with her weight control – and her food control!

Another client, Cynthia, a travel agent, has a history of abusing cookies. But she's able to keep them in her life without danger by *never* buying a bag for her home. Instead, she keeps a bag in her office, in a closet far away from her desk, where it's not in her line of vision or easy to reach. At night, she takes home two cookies – no more, no less – and enjoys them after dinner.

I do the same as Cynthia with my evening dessert, which features a Belgian waffle. When I kept a box at home, and I saw it every time I opened the freezer, I found I'd eat more waffles and continue to be tempted. I discovered, however, the perfect solution. I now keep a box in a freezer in my office, and when I want dessert I take home one waffle. I make strawberry shortcake by topping the waffle with a few strawberries and a swirl of fat-free aerosol cream.

It's my favourite dessert, and I eat it often with no weight gain – and no tug of war with temptation!

In a recent survey of men and women who lost weight and kept it off, it was reported that two out of three of the 'masters of weight control *keep problem foods out of their house and out of sight*'. Like my clients, these winners at long-term weight control have discovered the value of Box It In techniques.

When you're aware that a certain food can sabotage you, that it can be a double-edged sword between pleasure and pain, you will be more likely to stay alert to not abusing it. The strategy of Boxing It In lets you stay on the side of pleasure, by keeping your attention on your problem food. This is a great psychological advantage because *those who stay focused, stay trim*.

When you follow the new rules you've established for yourself, you turn off your automatic pilot for eating and become more selective, wise and careful in your food choices. Instead of randomly consuming at will, you can develop a personal strategy that will free you for the rest of your life from the snares that have repeatedly tripped you up. It's very empowering to set boundaries based on your own behaviour, lifestyle and history – and then to see the positive results in your life. When you consistently honour your new guidelines, you're sure to always be successful!

Eat and Be Merry

Many of my clients practice Boxing It In at holidays, family picnics or other special events. They give themselves the pleasure of eating cake on their birthday or sampling every dish on the holiday table.

Weight gain over the holiday season doesn't come from one feast. The danger is in the foods and the trays of baked goods left out in the office and at home in the days before and after the holidays as well as the leftovers. The secret to getting through these events in your life is to Box In special meals on the holiday itself, or the evening before, rather than to randomly eat whatever you see, whenever you see it, throughout the season.

It's really great news for my clients to realize that they don't have to give up the great dinners that mark their birthdays or other special events. Enjoying a fine meal is part of the celebration of life and a wise and appropriate use of food.

The Tale of a Southern Belle and the Pleasure of Pecan Pie

One of my clients, Suzanna, is from Atlanta. She lives in Idaho, now, but her tastes have stayed true to her roots. She loves Southern cooking.

When I first met her, she had many trigger foods. She got them all under control after a while, except for one – pecan pie. She was absolutely committed to staying in charge of her weight, and she did not want to resign herself to missing the enjoyment of this favourite rich dessert, so she found a solution that uses the Box It In technique of eating a favourite food only at a specified time.

She allows herself to eat as much pecan pie as she wants at two dinners when she returns to visit her family four times a year. She doesn't bake it the rest of the year, buy it, or order it in restaurants. She has moments of wanting it, but they pass swiftly. She doesn't mind waiting for the pleasure of her favourite nutty confection – and she's added a new meaning to the phrase: 'There's no place like home.'

Of course, it's still important to be prepared when facing a problem food. One of my clients, who has a particular fondness for pumpkin pie, has a creative plan that she follows when she's presented with it at occasions such as Thanksgiving. She enjoys every bite of the pumpkin pie filling, but leaves the crust behind. She's happy to do it, because it isn't the crust that makes the pie special. Every pie has a crust. It's the pumpkin filling that's her passion. With Box It In strategy, she can keep this favourite and unique taste in her life while avoiding the food that would sabotage her success at weight control.

Italian rum cake is a particular pleasure of mine, and I do some Boxing In with it. On Christmas day, I allow myself to eat as many slices as I want, knowing I won't be seeing rum cake again soon. Although I don't limit the quantity that I eat on this one day, I do limit the availability. This high-calorie treat won't be on my grocery list or appearing in my day-to-day life in the coming months, and that knowledge allows me to give myself the freedom for a delicious, special indulgence.

BOX IT IN OR OUT?

Maybe the food you love is crisps or ice cream or biscuits. Whatever it is, if you want it to remain in your life, you must take a good look at how, where and when it is least likely to be a problem for you. *Your lifelong success at weight control depends on how well you handle the foods that tempt you the most.*

All of us want to keep all the foods we love in our life, all of the time. But that is just not realistic in an adult world. When we grow up, we accept that we can't have everything we want. We recognize the need to set priorities and be selective.

Selectivity is a part of living at peace with ourselves, and personal happiness is living out the vision that we have for our lives. If your vision is to see yourself as a trim person for all the years to come, then you will know that your favourite size has to come before your favourite food. You'll understand that what is essential for happiness is not the same as what is simply nice to have or 'what looks interesting'.

Since you can't have it all, all the time, your guidelines need to be: how much can you have? Where and when? And what food management style works best for you? What choices will help you to be 'foodSmart?' – to spend your calories wisely?

With strategy, you can enjoy your favourite foods without putting on pounds. However, it works only if the food is indeed manageable. In certain cases, there may be a number or perhaps just one or two foods that can't be handled in this way because they trigger such powerful cravings in people with physiological hypersensitivities.

But the good news, the promise of the Box It In strategy is this: *anything that you love that you can truly control can be a part of your life forever.*

Use these three key techniques to guide you:

1. If you can have 'just a sliver' when it's served to you, but you would overeat it if you were in your home, then *only* eat it when you're a guest in someone's home or *only* in restaurants. And limit those occasions, too, to special events, or hold yourself to eating it in specified restaurants.

2. If you can Box In a food at home, be sure to keep it under 'wraps'. Cover tempting leftovers with foil – not in see-through plastic. Store them out of sight in the farthest reaches of the refrigerator, even hidden in the vegetable compartment. Keep other snacks and treats in closed cupboards, the more remote and inconvenient the better.

3. If you eat it compulsively when it's in the house, then *never* bring it home. If you buy it for yourself, limit the amount by choosing small packages and single-serving sizes – or throw out the extras in the package before you put it in your kitchen.

As I've suggested before, there may be a few foods for some of us that are not a good choice for Boxing In. They ignite such strong desires, they activate my F-Q principle – first you have a little, then the *frequency* increases and eventually, invariably, an increase in *quantity* follows. These foods trigger *ongoing cravings* and *obsessive thoughts* and lead you into a process that wears down your motivation to stay in charge. It's the pattern that you must break if you're going to be a lifelong winner at weight control.

As you consider your problem foods, you may conclude that it might be easier to Box Out one or two foods from your life. This is a critical choice, upon which your success hinges. *When you think historically and see that you have a long history of abuse with a certain food, that every time you've gone back to it, it's created powerful cravings and obsessive thoughts, and your weight has returned, then the key to control is realizing that the risk of eating it is not worth the momentary pleasure it may give.* It's far better to get a few foods out of your life – and still enjoy the figure that you want for life.

But how do you give up your favourite foods? Is it possible? Does it mean living with suffering, constant feelings of cravings and deprivation – feeling you're missing out on the fun? For most of my clients, the opposite has been true. They tell me repeatedly that their decision to Box Out a food has made their lives easier and their success at weight control far more certain. With the Box It Out techniques that follow, you'll discover how this wonderful outcome can be yours too.

As always, you must be truthful with yourself. As Henry David Thoreau observed: *It takes two to speak the truth – one to speak it, another to hear it.* Through the pages of this book, I'm sharing the truths I've learned, but you must be honest with yourself about how they apply to your life. Otherwise you'll be 'boxing yourself in' for a lifetime of weight problems.

Taking Control of a Food That Doesn't Work for You

For some people, when it comes to trigger foods, good intentions just aren't enough. You can know that Box It In is *not working* for you if any of these statements describe you:

- You think about a food more and more often even though you may be eating it regularly.
- Your cravings return or increase.
- You continually renegotiate the terms of the agreement you made with yourself so you can eat the food more often.
- When you stop or limit the food, you lose weight.
- When you return to eating it, you start gaining weight back.
- You break promises to yourself about how much or how often you'll consume it.

If you recognize these symptoms, don't kid yourself. Talking about 'just a little' or 'just this once' is the road back to fat. In such a situation, it's time to admit that a food doesn't work for you. It's time to Box It Out of your life.

It's important to understand that there is a considerable difference between doing without something of our own accord and being made to do without it. With this strategy, it is *not* that you *can't have* your favourite food or that anyone is taking it away from you, but that you are being honest with yourself. You are choosing to free yourself from weight problems, cravings and constant battles that wear you down. In a world full of life-threatening illness, starvation and homelessness, one food or type of food is never *really* a necessity – but it may be necessary to get it out of your life so you can have the life you want. Never lose your good values; most of the people living on this planet today have never spent a millisecond of their lives thinking about the food you think you can't live without.

One of the saddest lessons in my practice is that I've seen thousands of clients whose journey through a continuing series of weight failures mirrors the similar struggle of millions of people – those who have never succeeded on a weight programme because of just one or two foods. I've worked with many clients who were heavy in their 60s because of the very same foods that made them heavy in their 30s, 40s and 50s. How painful to realize that they would never have known one dieting failure after another had they simply Boxed Out one or two foods. They have spent decades being heavy – along with the physical and emotional costs – because of these foods! And one of the laments I hear most frequently in the clients who have successfully Boxed Out a food is: 'Why didn't I realize this sooner?'

In choosing to avoid a certain food, you are freeing yourself from constant weight problems, cravings and the unending battle with temptations that wear down your willpower.

This is what John Drybread had in mind when he wrote: *For those who are given to excess, abstinence is easier than moderation.*

Once a food is eliminated from your diet, you will be able to live with a new sense of freedom and control – and most of all success. My clients who have made a decision to Box Out a food have discovered one of the great secrets of weight control: *far from feeling deprived without a certain food, they felt liberated – from cravings and old struggles and from years of failure with their weight – and they find it's much easier to live without it.*

At one time, I made the mistake of thinking, perhaps as you may think, that it would be *harder* to eliminate a food than to eat it in moderation. But my clients' successes taught me that the opposite is true – *it's easier!*

Some of my clients, when they reached the maintenance level in their diets, would respond to my suggestion that they go back to a certain food with a horrified expression and an adamant 'No! Never!'

In making this adjustment, it's critical that you know how to outmanoeuvre your psyche's deprivation mechanism. Never say 'You can't have it.' It's not true, and it may trigger feelings of deprivation. Say to yourself instead, 'It doesn't work for me.' This way you don't fall into the 'Eve Complex' of something becoming more attractive because it's forbidden. You can have all you want, whenever you want. But if you do, you will never have the life or the control that you want. You are using your intelligence and freely choosing not to have it so you can choose to be trim.

'I don't miss it. It's easier if I don't begin,' they'd tell me again and again. 'It might reactivate my cravings. I'm afraid to go back.' Statements of this kind helped me understand how powerful it can be for some people to *not take a taste* of a food.

The same message kept coming back to me, and the lesson was clear: *to Box Out a food is one of the most powerful and surprisingly easy techniques for mastering cravings.*

My clients follow the same rule for high-carbohydrate items, such as pasta. Or they Box In the quantity of the food by ordering it as an appetizer, a small serving size.

In this way, they've been able to sample all the magnificent creations of the great chefs of the world – and emerge unscathed!

Instead of food items, they buy themselves beautiful clothes or other special souvenirs.

As I discuss in the Third Thin Commandment, The Problem May Be in the Food, Not in You, the reason you've been unable to moderate a food may have little or nothing to do with your willpower or strength of character. Certain foods trigger your appetite and overpower the appetite control centre in the brain. It may have to do with your own biological hypersensitivity to the taste, look or aroma of a certain food.

When a food is a part of life, it enhances life, but when it becomes the centrepiece of a human life – when it comes before your appearance and your control over your own body and subjects you to continuing failure at something that is so precious to your happiness and health, when it comes before your wardrobe, self-image and promises that you make to yourself – then that food does not enhance your life, but diminishes it! Eating such a food does not free you; it imprisons you – and sentences you to a lifelong struggle with your weight and with failure.

This is the change in thinking that is so important to understand: eating the food *is* the deprivation because it deprives you of reaching your critical life goals. And when you make this shift in your mind, you truly come to see a great new truth in a new light:

Boxing Out a food is not about deprivation, but about liberation.

The prevailing thinking in the professional diet field says we should give in and indulge cravings occasionally because too much deprivation sabotages weight loss, leads to bingeing and wears down resolve. You may have read many times that if you feel deprived, your diet will fail, but that's only half of the truth.

It's correct *if* you don't change your thinking. But it's *not true* when you realize that just one or two foods have stolen your figure, your favourite clothes size, and your success at managing your weight. It's not true when you understand that by *not* eating a certain food, you will actually be deactivating the craving mechanism within your brain and your psyche. You'll be turning off cravings forever. When you learn to say 'No, thank you' to a food *and* use the techniques of Box It Out, you'll discover, as so many of my clients have, that you will be saying 'yes' to being thin for life.

In her books *Thin for Life* and *Eating Thin for Life*, author Anne M. Fletcher, MS, RD, the noted nutritionist, studied 208 weight-loss masters who had lost at least 9 kg (20 lb) and kept them off for 3 or more years. She found that *more than half* of these people just avoid the foods they know will trigger overeating. Obviously these winners know that beginning with a little will lead to more and that *not even starting is the smart way to go.*

If a problem food has been in your life for years, if you've struggled with your weight every time you've tried to eat it in moderation, then you have the evidence that if you continue consuming it in the same way, you will never achieve success at weight control. As I've said before, the mark of smart people is that they avoid doing, again and again, what doesn't work.

GETTING RID OF A FOOD THAT'S SABOTAGED YOU, AGAIN AND AGAIN

What do you do about the chocolate chip cookies, nibble foods or other foods that always seem to be getting the better of you? Follow these guidelines for Boxing Out troublesome foods.

1. **Shift your thinking.** Living trim doesn't mean you have to give up the pleasure of fine dining or even most of your

favourite foods. By making a conscious choice to avoid one food or type of food, you know that you *can* eat it any time you want, but if you do, you would be *depriving yourself* of a lifetime of being thin, in control and free of cravings. Realize, also, that not eating this food will free up thousands or tens of thousands of calories per month to enjoy other foods you love.

2. **Set a date when you are going to stop eating it and reward yourself for the decision.** Buy yourself a present, such as a new outfit in a smaller size. Tell yourself you can have the food again, from a certain age on, such as 75.

3. **Tell yourself: it's not an option.** The human psyche is prone to negotiate boundaries where pleasure is involved, but when it hears an unequivocal 'No!' it becomes surprisingly obedient and respects the line.

4. **Remember to think historically.** Calorie counters say, 'What's wrong with a taste?' My clients and I know that's a big mistake. Taste buds don't care if they get a little bite or many big bites – once they're reactivated, they're back in control. After that, eating your trigger food is like throwing petrol on a fire. One taste can reactivate the craving memory of a lifetime. It's not about the calories but the cravings! Once you're struggling with cravings, weight control feels much harder. The size of the portion is irrelevant to the power of the cravings that will follow.

5. **Avoid eye contact.** No one ever graduated from baking school for turning out ugly looking biscuits, cakes and pastries. *No eye contact allowed* is a smart strategy.

6. **Don't allow thinking that sabotages you.** Don't tolerate an inner voice that speaks to you about your problem food. Avoid reading about it in recipes, magazines and restaurant reviews.

7. **Give up resentments and thinking 'It's not fair'.** Wayne W. Dyer, PhD, a leading therapist and bestselling author, counsels that when you are filled with resentments, you turn over control of your emotional life. But when you depersonalize an issue, you have no need to feel resentment, and you 'immu-

nize' yourself against negativity and doubt. Remember: the problem may be in the food, not in you, so it doesn't work for you – unless you want to wear it!

8. **Cut off food curiosity.** If you've given up desserts, there's no reason to ask for a menu 'just for a look'. If pasta is a problem for you, then don't study the pasta selections in a restaurant menu. You have no reason to give your problem food any role in your life.

9. **Make a public announcement about your food choices.** If you tell everyone at a party or at your table that you don't eat a certain food, you commit yourself to not eating it. The power of embarrassment is greater than willpower.

10. **Try not to buy it for your home or buy a substitute.** If you must buy it for other family members, select a small supply in single serving sizes. Or purchase a variety of the food that appeals to you the least. If you like Cherry Garcia ice cream, buy another flavour for the family that doesn't tempt you. (Not keeping it in your immediate environment permanently is the most helpful strategy of all. That's what the winners strive to do.)

11. **Reinforce your commitment with the single most powerful statement that supports your resolve: I don't begin; I don't have any problem.** This is what almost all of my clients say when they see their Boxed Out food. It cuts off thinking and debating. For some, I have qualified the phrase: *if I don't take the first little taste, I don't begin. I don't have a problem*, since I found that the negotiators among us could often get into trouble by saying to themselves, *I won't begin, but I'll just have a little taste.* But, of course, having a little taste is indeed beginning. As I have noted, *the size of the portion is irrelevant to the power of the cravings that will follow* – not to mention the reawakening of the interest in and the thinking about the food again.

12. **Reward yourself.** Replace the 'food treat' psychology of your childhood with the adult reward system of a new outfit, a magazine, or something special you want. You deserve rewards, and being trim will be one of them.

You may think that it's endlessly difficult to refuse a food you've always loved, but with smart strategy, the once seemingly impossible becomes possible – even easy. The truth is that cravings fade over time if they're not reinforced through tasting and other visual cues. And once you make a decision to give up a food because it doesn't work for you, life becomes simpler. When you've made a clear choice, within a short time, your psyche will accept the change, and you'll stop thinking about the food that once occupied so much of your thoughts.

Dr Dean Ornish, the director of the Preventive Medicine Research Institute and the author of four bestselling books about diet and health, has come to a similar conclusion. *Despite conventional wisdom, he writes, it is actually easier to make big changes in diet all at once than to make small, gradual ones…Most people find that they feel so much better so quickly that the choices become clearer and worth making…to increase the joy of living.*

SUBSTITUTION IS OFTEN THE KEY TO SUCCESS

My client, Annette, remains untroubled when buying cakes and biscuits for her husband and children, although she has Boxed Out products made with white flour, fat and sugar. She shrewdly chooses varieties that are made with raisins and nuts, which have no appeal

When You Can't Remove a Food from Sight

Many people find that they can say 'no' to a food for a short time, but if they sit with it, whether it's a bread-basket or a tray of cakes, it soon starts to wear down their resolve.

My client, Matthew, a lawyer, frequently dines out with clients. Since he can't avoid eye contact with the breadbasket, his Boxed Out food, he uses the clever strategy of announcing at the beginning of the meal that the rolls look delicious, but there's no way he can eat any.

'It works every time,' he tells me. 'Once I've identified myself as a non-bread eater, I know I'll be embarrassed if I contradict myself. So I'm not tempted.'

for her. Another client, whose family likes pastries, buys them pastries filled with whipped cream, which she dislikes. These women know how to strategize!

What to Do When You're Falling Out of Control

Even the most successful weight strategist can hit a rough patch sometime. If you find yourself suddenly falling into constantly overeating, your control is slipping, and you may even be bingeing. These crisis-intervention techniques may help stop your slide:

1. **Remember the lesson of The Fourth Thin Commandment, 'Structure Gives Control'.** Immediately write out an eating plan for the next 24 hours, several days, a week, or longer. The further you can plan ahead, the more the strategy can help put you back in charge.

2. **Make it easy to do the right thing.** Remove from your home any foods that are a temptation for you. Watch out for products that might not have been a problem before but may now have a new appeal.

3. **Don't turn a detour into a catastrophe.** Turn off the thinking that suggests that because you've gone overboard, you're out of control and you might as well continue overeating.

4. **Fight the temptation to eat too little.** Many people, when they feel they've consumed too many calories in one day, will go too far in the other direction for the next day or two. They'll undereat, which leaves them hungry and more prone to losing control. Avoid this common mistake by eating healthy meals and snacks every 3 to 4 hours throughout the day.

5. **If you've gone back to a trigger food, especially sweets and/or a flour and sugar product, and you've reactivated cravings and recurring thoughts about it, you can address the problem by 'throwing protein at it'.** This tactic isn't well supported in current diet thinking, but I've found that a diet, for a day or two, that consists of as many as four to five small meals that contain a good source of low-fat protein will stabilize blood-sugar levels and reduce strong cravings as well as any increased appetite. If you've been eating too much creamy ice cream, for

THE MORE YOU EAT, THE MORE YOU CRAVE

If you're hypersensitive to food containing sugar, flour or fat, or those that have a crunchy texture, having a little of it doesn't help,

instance, the substitute of a creamy, cold dilled egg salad (see my recipe on page 237) may jump-start you back on track with a healthy eating plan. I'm not suggesting this as an everyday technique, but as a strategy to turn to when you're feeling especially vulnerable. You might even overeat protein a bit to be sure your blood-sugar levels remain even.

6. **If you're continuing to crave sugar, try saturating your taste buds with salty, spicy or hot food.** Pickles, salsas and other hot sauces may reduce your cravings. You might also try a sugar substitute in liquid form, which most people are less likely to abuse, such as diet drinks or shakes.

7. **If you've been overindulging in salty foods, such as nuts or potato crisps, try pickles to knock out your cravings, or my 'fried' courgette sticks or chips (see my recipe on page 235).**

8. **Sometimes eating isn't about food. You may be upset, angry or hurt. Talk it over with a friend or counsellor, or keep a journal.** Once you express your feelings in speech or writing, they're out and they become easier to manage in appropriate ways. By simply venting emotions, you increase the likelihood of immediately returning to control.

Your situation might also be the result of a change in your attitude. Perhaps you're pleased with what you weigh, you may have recently dropped a number of pounds and you've lost some of your motivation to be careful with your diet. In such a case, it's important to make a decision that you won't allow yourself to become sloppy with your eating habits.

Remember the advice I've given you to *get the mood out of the food*. Take back your power. Don't allow other people or external events to control what you put into your body. Refuse to eat a single extra calorie because of the negative people who may be in your life.

and it may hurt. As I've discussed, these ingredients – as well as some others – can actually overpower the appetite control centre and change the brain's neurochemistry. You can come to constantly crave sweet baked goods or other products to the exclusion of alternative foods.

But if you cut out these foods and use the strategies to Box It Out, the cravings will begin to weaken and eventually go away. And there's more great news: one of the major findings of my work is that when you eliminate the handful of foods that tempt you the most, your appetite for all foods seems to fall significantly as well as your interest in them. It may be due to cutting back on the level of carbohydrates or simply diminishing temptation, but whatever the mechanism, you have much less hunger- and food-obsessed thinking and much greater success with your weight control. The majority of my clients have discovered that they no longer crave or think about their former problem food, and they're only tempted by it if they happen to see or be seated near it for some length of time. Even then, the craving is no longer an overwhelming compulsion, but just a mild feeling.

DON'T FORGET TO REWARD YOURSELF

Another characteristic of the human psyche, one of the strongest, is that it likes to be given special acknowledgement with treats and presents. I encourage my clients to celebrate their success with weight control by indulging in any luxury that would make them happy.

I also tell them that now that they've grown up, they need to choose adult gifts for themselves. Children are rewarded with sweets, a grown-up deserves presents that enhance life much more significantly.

When you're pleased with yourself and proud of how you look, a trip to a tropical paradise or just a visit to the local beach or swimming pool can give you a chance to look great in shorts or your swimsuit. It can do wonders for your self-esteem. It's especially satisfying to buy new clothing in your favourite size, and the pleasure strengthens your commitment to continue following The Thin Commandments, which are your ticket to a lifetime of being trim.

One of my clients, an executive at a financial management company, understood the power that the right purchase could harness for keeping up his motivation. He bought himself a sports car. 'Even if I bought myself the most expensive suit I could find, I still might let myself slip and gain back some weight,' he explained to me. 'But I know I'll never let myself become so fat again that I couldn't fit into my great car. It was worth every penny because it guarantees that I will always be thin. Every time I drive it, I'm reminded of how much I want to live this life that I have worked so hard to earn.'

Box It In and Box It Out can bring success to you, too. With these powerful strategies, you and you alone decide what foods you can and cannot control. You choose the foods that you will abstain from, limit or continue to eat when you like based on your food history, sensitivities and preferences. When you're in charge, when you have a vision of yourself as a trim person, when you know what is important to you, and you set the boundaries that work to help you reach your goals, you become a winner at weight control. You gain freedom forever from food struggles – and a lifelong assurance of living thin.

Guilt doesn't burn a single calorie, but learning from mistakes can save you thousands.

The Seventh Thin Commandment:
Slips Should Teach You, Not Defeat You

COMMANDMENT ESSENTIALS

- Error control is the essence of weight control.
- Don't say 'I blew it' if you make an eating mistake.
- Don't undereat in an attempt to compensate for cheating the previous day.
- Discover your predictable pattern in eating mistakes.
- Use binge-busters to end a craving.
- Don't go hungry.
- Find something to do, such as reading a book or knitting, to help get your mind off your craving.
- Think substitution, not deprivation.
- Put a negative association with the foods that tempt you most.

WOULDN'T IT BE GREAT IF THERE were just one thing that made you a winner at weight control? There is.

One characteristic marks every winner I've worked with and eludes everyone who doesn't succeed: those who master weight control learn from their mistakes instead of losing to them.

You may think that winners make fewer mistakes, that they're a different breed of human. The truth is they're not. They're just like you. They make mistakes. *It's how they deal with their mistakes* that makes them winners. They treat a diet slip like any human error. They cut it off, see what went wrong and take steps to prevent it from happening again. *Winners deal with mistakes by learning from them; failures deal with mistakes by blindly repeating them!*

Errors can slow your progress and weaken your focus. *Our goal is to prevent error, not promote it.* However, this book is designed to meet the needs of how real people behave in the real world as opposed to a perfect one. Human beings make mistakes. 'To err is human.'

But did you ever think you could make mistakes and *still lose weight* – in fact, lose all the weight you want? With the right skills, you can. Very few of my clients have perfect weeks, but almost all of them lose weight!

You will make mistakes – this is certain. But equally certain is that *these errors do not have to lead to weight gain, but in fact can lead to you being a master at stopping them quickly and keeping them at bay in the future. There can be no success at weight control without successful error control!*

Past mistakes do *not* mean future failure.

Charles was a successful architect but had failed on so many diets that he didn't think I could help much. 'How long have you been trying?' I asked.

'Thirty-plus years,' he said. 'Just like my parents, a new diet every couple of months. I guess it's in my genes.'

Maybe there's something of Charles in some of you, readers. You've tried many times over the years to lose weight and just as many times not succeeded. Maybe you, too, had heavy parents and feel genetics can't be overcome. The good news is that none of these suspicions is true, and the fact that you are reading this proves that you somehow suspect this!

THE SINGLE BIGGEST MISTAKE

I told Charles that just the fact that he came to me proved that he still believed he could win the game of weight control. 'I always believe at first,' he said, 'but then something happens, and I blow the whole thing. I don't really see what you can do to stop that.'

I told him he was right about one thing: I couldn't stop him from sooner or later making an error on his diet, because everyone makes mistakes! 'In fact,' I said, 'I'm sure I make more mistakes than many of my clients! But what I can help you with is *how you learn from your mistakes.* That's what will make the difference this time! There's just one mistake you have to promise you'll never make again.'

'Which one?' he asked.

'Just promise me – and more important, promise yourself – *that you'll never again say, "I blew it".'*

He looked shocked. 'Just never say, "I blew it"?'

'Or any of its familiar variants: "I blew the day. The day is ruined. It's all over." That's the only real mistake that leads to failure in weight control. Everything else will be your learning laboratory.'

He smiled and said, 'It's a deal.'

That deal helped Charles lose 29 kg (65 lb) over the following months!

A few years later, I saw his picture in the newspaper, still looking very trim, at the dedication of a building he designed. I called him to congratulate him. We talked a bit and then he said, 'You know, Doctor, I still have never made that great mistake!'

I paused because it had been a while – I wasn't sure what mistake he meant.

'The single biggest mistake!' he quickly filled me in. 'Ever since the first time we met in your office, I never once have said, "I blew the day"!'

THE BIGGEST CAUSE OF EXCESS POUNDS IS *NOT* A FOOD

It's not even a behaviour – it's a *mindset.* It's a mental habit that reacts to a diet slip by giving up, 'letting the screen go blank'. When dieters cheat (eat a high-calorie dessert, say), this one error tends to become a reason to stop *all* their efforts at weight control. Instead of handling it like any human error – asking, 'What can I learn from this?' – they say, 'Well, I blew it, I might as well blow the rest of the day (or the weekend, or longer).'

This 'I blew it' syndrome is different from the momentary *feeling* of 'I blew it', which we all may get after eating too much. Winners certainly have experienced this *feeling* with regard to a particular meal or food. But then they become more careful and balance the excess with smart eating. *The failures say, 'I blew it', and let their mental screens go blank. Their eating gets careless, and this carelessness engulfs the day and often the next day(s). This is the 'I blew it' syndrome.* Something in you says that you might as well eat all you can for the rest of the day so you can *'get it all in' before going back on your diet. I also call this 'the last meal syndrome'* and tell my clients: 'It will never be your last meal. You're not being thrown in the dungeon. There will be too much food in your life, never too little. So don't act as if a great famine is about to start.' The good news, though, is that these mistakes can easily be contained, using the techniques in this book.

One of the great lessons in my work is how many people approach weight control with the idea 'I'll either be perfect or perfectly horrible.' They don't think this way when they learn any other skill, such as knitting, driving, using their software, or even parenting.

Of course, the motive for weight loss is often so strong that most people *do* start a weight programme perfectly. They're in what I call the 'weight-loss zone', just to see the numbers come down. This is why people can give up food entirely and start out with just liquid protein drinks. When you're miserable because you don't fit into your clothes, doing any diet brings relief, even if you feel that you're swimming underwater, holding your breath to do it perfectly. But as the weight comes off, and the clothes get loose and the compliments start, experience has shown that sooner or later you'll have to come up for 'error'.

And when you do make a mistake – as we all do – *don't continue and make the fatal mistake of saying 'I blew the day'*. Because this syndrome is *the* dividing line between those who lose weight only to gain it back and those who keep it off forever!

Why the 'I Blew It' Syndrome Is Terminal to Diets

Let's get one thing straight: *no one ever gets heavy from one mistake, one meal of extra calories, a bag of sweets or even several hors d'oeuvres at a cocktail party! It's only when you lose control of the eating that comes after the mistake that the weight gain begins.*

The 'I blew it' syndrome:

- Sets up an impossible tension in your life – that you have to be either perfect or a failure
- Lets your mental screen go blank, so you shut down everything that you've learned about food management
- Lets mistakes pile up, which drowns your motivation, skews your perspective and overwhelms your willpower
- Destroys focus on your eating and weight control. (Studies all show that staying *focused* on your eating behaviour is what makes you a winner.)
- Is self-defeating. It cuts off learning from the mistake and locks you into a pattern of repeating it
- Only helps you learn that you're gaining weight, which is obvious
- Ruins your chance to cut off the mistake and keep any weight gain small and temporary
- Keeps you from proving to yourself that you *can* stop and correct the error, a tremendous source of empowerment
- Turns a few minutes of unwise eating into something that will take days, months or even years to make up for. It's not time efficient
- Paralyses you into a mode of helplessness that lets one mistake end up becoming thousands of calories
- Doesn't do justice to your intelligence
- Doesn't make you lose weight; it only makes you lose hope. Cutting off the error does the opposite – it builds hope and gives you power
- Doesn't answer the most important question of all: *what went wrong in this situation, and what could I do differently?*

ERROR CONTROL IS THE ESSENCE OF WEIGHT CONTROL

Erica was a struggling actress who was 'tired of playing the fat jolly friend of the romantic lead'. She apologized for crying, but she felt that she was wasting the years of her youth with failure after failure in weight control. I handed her a box of tissues and said, 'Erica, those years were anything but wasted. There are patterns and reasons why you've failed, and from those lessons, you can script a new future. That experience can show you just what you need to do to get the weight you want.'

She wiped her eyes and sighed. 'It just seems no matter how hard I try, ice cream defeats me!' I had to laugh, and she smiled. 'Erica, food has no IQ.'

'Maybe not, but there's something in me that has to have Rocky Road!'

'Do you really think your eating mistakes result from demonic possession?'

She burst out laughing and said, 'Well I did grow up in the Dakota!' (The Dakota is the New York City building where they filmed the movie *Rosemary's Baby.*) Then she sighed again and said, 'I just feel like a complete failure.'

'If food is winning against us, it doesn't mean we're weak, pathetic souls beyond redemption. It just means we have to figure out a better strategy. Most people who get into trouble with weight control haven't really failed, they've failed to plan. Error control is the basis of that plan. You've just never had a strategy for error control. You're certainly not a complete failure!'

Erica's beautiful eyes had turned serious. 'I never thought of that before,' she commented.

'Error control is one of the most neglected areas in my field, but I've found it to be the essence of weight control. Think about it. What weight-control programme is known for its strong emphasis on error-control techniques?'

'None that I've heard of,' she said. 'This makes so much sense to me!'

Erica was one of my clients who realized from the start that this particular thin commandment was the ultimate shortcut! The phrase 'I blew it' would never cross her lips. You could see her determination when she talked about a slip she made, eager to learn all she could from it!

Because she made this commandment her number one priority, Erica reached her desired weight as fast as any client I've ever had in her weight-control category. Error control is the essence of weight control. Letting your slips teach you and not defeat you goes to the heart of the weight problem. This commandment cuts across all the others because in following any of them (just like the real

Ten Commandments), people make mistakes. So knowing how to control and learn from mistakes makes any commandment work more powerfully.

The Magic Bullet for Error Control

The first thing to do after making a mistake is to stop it as soon as you can. Contain the mistake before it turns into an overwhelming series of mistakes. Just as there are chain smokers, there are 'chain eaters'. Don't allow the chain to start, and you will succeed in weight control!

As soon as you finish eating the improper food or conclude the overeating episode, talk to yourself in a new way. *Instead of saying, 'I blew it', say, 'Stop now'.* This breaks the 'I blew it' syndrome instead of allowing you to keep eating as if your diet had just been proven useless. It hasn't at all! The overwhelming majority of my clients who have made one or two errors during the week but cut them off quickly still lost weight. If you stop the mistake before it turns into a chain, you can still lose some weight for the week and never gain it back!

That's why it's so important to change your self-talk after an eating mistake. You have to change your thinking in order to change your weight permanently! Instead of telling yourself, 'I blew it', remember that failure (or even weight gain) doesn't come from one mistake but from 'letting your screen go blank' and letting a 1-minute mistake multiply into a calorie mountain that crushes your diet. Tell yourself 'Stop now', and don't start chain-eating, the deadliest threat to a diet I've found in all my years of work.

The longer you persist in your eating mistake – the more chain-eating you do – the harder it will be to get back on track. And by then you're making other mistakes, and you feel like you're just sinking deeper and deeper. So it's immensely important to have a strategy to contain the mistake before it turns into chain-eating.

THE 24-HOUR SECRET

In the course of helping thousands of people in their struggle not to chain-eat, one day it struck me that they all had something in common, a tendency not shown by winners: most people who make a diet mistake will continue the pattern for the rest of the day! *I call it the 'slip to sleep' syndrome.*

So know the following, and you can take steps to avoid it: if you cheat on your diet, you will be strongly tempted to cheat more and more for the rest of the day and often for the next 24 hours. If you make a conscious, focused effort not to fall into the pattern for the rest of the day and into the next, the temptation to cheat passes. With good strategy, you can immediately cut it off! You can get through this manageable period of time and make the cheating an isolated event. You end the cycle of bingeing from day to day, avert chain-eating and do not gain weight from your slips. And that is the 24-Hour Secret.

From Slip to Sleep: The Critical Period

The essence of weight control is error control, and *the essence of error control is managing the period from slip to sleep.* If you have success in this short but crucial period, you will have success in getting to your optimal weight. In a very real sense, being a winner at weight control all boils down to this section, these words you are reading right now.

You're especially vulnerable from the time of your error to the time you go to bed. Most people tend to blow off the rest of the day, and often this spills into the next. *The battle of weight gain is won or lost in this critical period.*

Here's the core strategy my clients have found works best during this time.

• **Write out what you will eat for the rest of the day –
meals as well as snacks.** This is the most successful strategy. Push yourself; force yourself to make this menu. Remember the Nike commercial, and 'Just do it'. Rally your energy for this one small step, and make a giant leap toward mastering your error. Take care to pick healthy foods you like, so you won't end up feeling deprived.

• **Write out tomorrow's menu as well.** And make sure the right foods will be available.

• **Do a brief mental rehearsal.** This technique – which I explain at the end of this chapter (see page 140) – will desensitize you to the power of any tempting food *before* you even encounter it.

• **Use diversion.** Plan some interesting activity for the rest of the day. Anything that occupies the mind will quickly divert it from thoughts about food and cravings. *Avoid boredom at all costs!* When you're bored, the thought of food seems extra interesting – not because you're hungry but just because it might 'fill up' the empty time. The diversion may be as simple as making a few telephone calls or just staying busy with personal projects.

• **Commit to the menu you've written, from that point until you go to bed.** It's only a matter of hours. Anyone can comply.

Dealing with the 'Day-After' Syndrome

The day after a slip is easier, but it still has dangers. First: *be aware when you wake up that there is such a thing as the 'Day-After Syndrome' so you'll be prepared.* You may find a heightened interest in your cheat food because the memory of its taste is still vivid. Your taste-bud memory has been strongly reinforced – particularly if your error food was a simple carbohydrate such as sugar or a white-flour product. Tell yourself: *it's not an option.* But also tell yourself that your interest in these foods will decline over the course of the day as your blood sugar evens out. You won't crave them forever, just a few more hours.

Here's the best strategy for the 'Day-After Syndrome':

Start the day with exercise. Do *any* kind of exercise, even if it's for only 15 minutes. It's not just about burning calories; it's about *a healthy mindset.* It gives structure to your day, starts it with a positive commitment, and sets your mental focus to be careful and good to your body all day.

Go over your menu for the day. Make sure it's written out in advance and includes snacks and meals. *Pick only foods you like so you won't feel deprived!* The 'day after' is not a good time to trigger that other PMS – the 'Poor Me Syndrome'. Choose foods you like, even if they have more calories, so a feeling of deprivation won't tempt you to repeat the errors of yesterday.

Don't undereat! This should be your most important goal today. *Do not attempt to undereat to compensate for yesterday.* This can end up making you too hungry on a day when the cravings may already be stronger than usual. *It's not about losing weight the next day;*

it's about not losing ground. The key is rebuilding control and stop-ping the error pattern. Even if your scales are up a little – don't panic. Probably most of this gain is water retention from salt and carbohydrate intake and will be gone tomorrow with proper eating. Avoid the scales entirely if it will cause too much negativity.

Have a fourth meal. A fourth meal of low-calorie, low-fat protein keeps blood sugar at an optimal level. Stabilized blood sugar puts off your hunger and significantly reduces cravings. Schedule it on your menu for when you're most vulnerable (late afternoon for most people).

Use visualization. See yourself eating the proper meals and snacks you've written on your menu. And try this ultimate visual-ization: put an article of clothing you love but is still too tight to wear where you'll see it during the day.

Reduce temptation. Don't go to restaurants you know are danger zones, and avoid food shopping if you can. Get rid of any leftovers or give them away. And try not to look at foods that aren't on your menu.

Reach out and keep busy. Catch up on overdue phone calls to upbeat people you like. The goal here is the same as from slip to sleep: do something enjoyable to kill boredom and *block* food thoughts. If you don't want to talk to someone, try an enjoyable activity instead. Reaching out redirects the mind to one of the most interesting, fulfilling acts – connecting with another person you care about or a rewarding activity, *not* food.

I have found that the vast majority of overeaters can break the 'I blew it' syndrome by using these strategies. And almost invariably, my clients who cut off mistakes this way for 24 hours don't gain a pound and typically go on to lose weight that week.

And even more important, they've learned how to stop chain-eating, a major enemy of thin – not just for when they're losing the weight, but for the rest of their lives.

All it takes for most people is to use this technique three or four times! By then you'll find that saying 'I blew it' is no longer automatic, but getting back on track is!

The biggest surprise is that this pattern, which has doomed so many to failure for so long, can be broken quickly – with the right strategy. Try it!

KNOW YOUR PATTERN AND YOU CAN PREDICT YOUR BEHAVIOUR

Once you have contained your mistake, it's time to learn from it. As we note many times in this book, there is an amazing amount of predictability in eating behaviour. If you know your pattern, you can predict your behaviour and develop a plan to control it for the future. And I have learned time and again in my work: *errors almost always follow a typical pattern*. The same people gain back the same weight with the same foods in the same place at the same time of day (or week) for the same reasons they gave themselves the last time they slipped! It's like Yogi Berra famously said, 'It's *déjà vu* all over again.'

Look for a pattern. That's number one. I say there is a pattern. You'd be surprised how many clients say there isn't, but after they review the following questions, they smile and say, 'Oh, *that!*'

Unlock Your REP (Repeating Eating Pattern)

These questions uncover *your* predictable pattern in eating mistakes. This pattern is important to learn so you can plan the right preventive strategies.

What type of *food?* Was it a sweet or crunchy food? Creamy? A baked item? What food was it exactly that started you off? Do you have a history of abusing a particular food?

What type of *mood?* What kind of state were you in when you made the mistake – nervous, sleep-deprived, bored, stressed, angry, frustrated? Did you tell yourself you were hungry? What reason did you give yourself?

What *environment?* What *place* were you in when you made the mistake? Were you in a restaurant? At the movies, outdoors, a friend's house, your mother's – or was it in your own home? If so, in what room? The kitchen, the dining room, or in front of the TV? Or were you in the office? This is a problematic place for many of us. Unlike at home, you can't control what foods are brought into your place of work. Holiday seasons, grateful clients, conference food, vending machines, the office cafeteria – work tempts you with food you've made a full-time job of keeping out of your home!

What *people* **were you with?** Were you with anyone when your eating went wrong? Friends? Business associates? Family? Also ask: were you with a large group of people? Studies have shown that *people tend to eat much more with a large group* than when alone or one-on-one. This will alert you to be prepared by eating something before you go out for group meals so you will be less tempted by everyone else's food or by being hungry.

What *time* **was it?** One of the most reliable truths in my work is that eating mistakes have a favoured *time of day*. This is what I called the 'Cinderella Syndrome' earlier in the book. Knowing when the clock strikes for *you* tells you when it's time to take preventive measures. And also take a look at the *time of the week*. Is *your* Friday Night Fight with heavyweight calories? Do Sunday night blues make you eat more?

10 NO-FAIL STRATEGIES TO PREVENT YOUR EATING MISTAKES

After containing your mistake and finding its pattern, it's time to *work out a strategy to stop it from repeating*. By avoiding the guilt of 'I blew it', you've reached this new stage of growth: where you use your slip as a compass to lead you to greater control and success. *Preventing* mistakes is infinitely better than rehabilitation! Successful preventive strategies save you great amounts of energy, frustration and time.

Strategy No. 1: Break availability. You can't eat what's not there! All studies show *the more food around; the more food you eat* – and the more you think of food and feel yourself tempted.

- If the 'cheat' food is around, get rid of it for the next week(s), even if it hasn't been bothering you.
- If it's for others in your family, *avoid proximity*. Stay away from it. If it's in the office, keep your distance.
- Don't work or have a phone chat in the 'Fat Room' (your kitchen).
- Avoid eye contact. Never underestimate the power of the visual! Just seeing some foods makes you want to put them right into your mouth. Put them in a paper bag instead or in

foil so when you open the refrigerator, the sight of them is unavailable to your eyes. Or put them on a high shelf in a cupboard with wooden doors. Take it from its see-through wrapping, and put it in a metal container. In a restaurant, don't 'eye' the whole menu, especially not the dessert section.

Strategy No. 2: Delay. Time is your friend if you're employing strategy. As time passes, cravings pass or other events capture your attention. If you tell yourself you'll eat the fattening food tonight or tomorrow instead of now, most typically when that time comes, you'll have a lot less interest in it. The original desire has usually dissipated.

Strategy No. 3: Use binge busters. Sometimes you want to end a craving immediately. That's where these easy-to-carry products come in handy.

- **Sugar Blocker Gum.** This gum is the most effective craving killer. It deactivates the sweet receptors on the tongue. After chewing for 10 minutes, anything sweet that you eat will no longer have a sweet taste, but rather, an unpleasant taste. And anything else you eat for the next half hour has very little or a bitter taste. Some of my clients who don't even like sweets use this gum because the unpleasant taste it creates in the mouth kills all cravings and appetite so you have no desire to eat. (At present this gum is widely available in the US but in other countries it can only be sourced via the Internet.)
- **Halls Sugar-Free Mentho-Lyptus drops.** These mentholated cough drops can be found in almost any chemist in the world. Just one overwhelms your taste buds and sense of smell. Walk into a room with pizza, and it won't have the same tempting aroma. Even the sight of it won't be appealing. There is no 5-minute wait with these drops, so when you need instant help, reach for these.
- **Listerine Breath Strips (or a comparable brand).** These flavoured breath strips melt on your tongue, are very easy to find and act immediately. They may or may not be stronger for you than the Halls drops. The key is to buy whichever has the sharpest taste for you and kills the desire to eat. Many of my clients put one or two of these on their tongue while they wait for their food in a restaurant, so they don't touch

the breadbasket, or they use them to kill a craving anytime they feel tempted or hungry.

Strategy No. 4: Don't go hungry. Success on a diet is not about being hungry. Getting hungry is usually not related to proper diet but to poor planning. But don't confuse hunger with boredom or listlessness or the 'habit hunger' you feel doing something you traditionally associate with eating, such as watching TV. Genuine hunger usually starts when you are approaching 3 to 4 hours without eating a healthy snack or meal. Here are six surefire strategies winners use to not go hungry.

- **Flood your appetite.** Most people don't gain weight from low-calorie *liquid* foods. Nor do they get compulsive about them. For something sweet, have a low-cal sweet *beverage*. A protein shake kills appetite and sugar cravings and is nutritious (make sure it's less than 100 calories). A low-calorie chocolate drink also works well.

  Carbonated beverages also kill hunger. Carbonation creates a feeling of fullness in the stomach. And typically, carbonated products are cold liquids. The combination of carbonation plus the cold makes a doubly strong appetite suppressor.

  Tomato juice is the ultimate hunger killer because it's a very heavy liquid and typically very flavourful. It's particularly helpful when you're asked at a restaurant if you'd like to order a drink. It's a safe appetite suppressant with very few calories – far less than alcohol or the contents of the breadbasket! For those who like spicy beverages, add a dash of Tabasco to your tomato juice. Some supermarkets also sell large bottles of spiced tomato juice.

- **Use temperature control for appetite control.** Extremes of temperature – hot or cold, particularly liquids – make the body feel full immediately and put off feelings of hunger. Try this experiment yourself: drink two glasses of water, one iced and the other room temperature. You'll find it takes much longer to finish the ice water, and it makes you feel fuller. As many people have discovered, when there's little time to eat, a cup of hot coffee does wonders to take the edge off your appetite. It'll even save you from picking on the breadbasket when hungry.

Most people would rank *soup* as number one in fixing their appetite. Have a bowl of tinned low-calorie vegetable soup. Carry around the instant soups that come in envelopes, such as Cup-a-Soup (especially the tomato!) or Slim-a-Soup.

• **Use your binge busters!** Halls Mentho-Lyptus drops, especially, make a powerful appetite killer. But Sugar Blocker Gum and breath strips (such as Listerine) also are reliable hunger stoppers.

• **Eat *the* appetite control cracker.** One cracker has a special place in my armament of anti-hunger weapons. I have seen more people abuse crackers than be helped by them, particularly the thin, salty, crispy ones. Most have too many carbohydrates and too little fibre. There is one notable exception – the *GG Scandinavian Bran Crispbread*. Only 18 calories and 3 grams of carbohydrates, but a generous 3 grams of fibre. And when you subtract the 3 grams of fibre from the 3 grams of carbohydrates, you get zero net carbs! It's the ultimate 'no-carb carb'. Two or three of these crackers kill appetite for hours with negligible calories even if you eat several extra throughout the day. All of my clients who use them daily say they are rarely hungry. They're not widely available in supermarkets but many health food shops stock them. They make great sandwiches with rich fibre, and you can carry them everywhere, so hunger will never again be part of your weight control. And you can search every health food shop there is and not find a cracker this thick and crunchy with those low calories and carbs.

My winners carry it everywhere in their briefcases or handbags for a snack or mini-meal. Turn it into a pizza with low-fat tomato sauce and a thin slice of light mozzarella; or a dessert with Quark cheese topped with jam or apple sauce (I'll talk about this further in the diet chapter).

The GG cracker is perfect for people who travel a lot and have irregular hours. Add it to your ThinPack: a self-sealing bag that also contains a low-cal hot chocolate, a low-cal Cup-a-Soup, and Laughing Cow Light Cheese triangles (which can last a few hours without refrigeration). Carry it with you, or put it in your glove compartment. It's particularly helpful for PMS hunger.

- **Throw veggies at it!** 'Think green and white.' Under my programme, most green and white vegetables made without fat are free foods. Make yourself half a pound of steamed broccoli with garlic, herbs and spices. Order steamed Chinese vegetables with spring onions and ginger. You can eat all you want.

- **Throw protein at it!** Pick a low-fat, nutritious protein, such as an egg-white omelette, grilled prawn salad, or my egg salad recipe (see page 237).

Strategy No. 5: Avoid packaging temptation. The colours, wording and photographs on all food packages have one goal only: to tempt you and increase your hunger for the product. Store packaged foods in brown bags to stop this temptation. Or discard the package entirely and put the food in an opaque container.

The best way to avoid the temptation of packaging you find especially alluring is to not even go down their aisles in the store, or at least don't stop when you do. And try not to shop in that vulnerable period of late afternoon when the blood sugar dips, or the packaging will look even more tempting. Or should I say *too* tempting?

Strategy No. 6: Use blocking behaviours. In psychology, the technique called *blocking behaviour* is the strategy of doing something *harmless* or positive to make it hard to do some other thing that is *harmful* or negative. This works very well for weight control. For example, at a party, my female winners will carry a clutch bag in one hand and a nonalcoholic drink in the other, stopping their hands from reaching out when fattening hors d'oeuvres come by.

Or if junk food is a problem when you turn on TV, block this behaviour with a no-eating rule, keep your hands busy with beverages, or chew on gum. Or instead of nuts or crisps, dip into a bowl of crunchy vegetables or roasted ones with spices. Many of my clients take up needlepoint or knitting to keep from eating when they watch TV. If you tend to 'pick' while cooking, put veggies on the worktop to nibble or sip on an ice-cold beverage with a straw. Or block that behaviour entirely by brushing your teeth and leaving a little toothpaste in your mouth. You could even pop a Halls Mentho-Lyptus drop or Listerine Breath Strip. (I suggest you always keep one or both of these items readily available in the kitchen or the room you use for preparing food.) You can block the negative behaviour or even convert it to a positive by eating healthy instead of fattening!

Strategy No. 7: Diversion. As talked about previously in this book, *diversion* is a powerful way of getting your mind off your craving by doing an activity you find absorbing or beneficial.

Strategy No. 8: Cognitive switching. *Cognitive switching* means talking to yourself in a new way.

All of us carry on a continuing internal dialogue about other people or events or about ourselves. How we talk to ourselves about *food* either encourages overeating or empowers us to limit or avoid it entirely. The winners at weight control permanently change their

What the Winners Say

When you first begin trying cognitive switching, it might seem artificial, and you have to push yourself to do it. But after a couple of days, it will become as natural for you as it has for my own clients. Think like a winner to cut off and prevent errors.

The food looks so tempting. Do I like it enough to wear it? I've tasted it all before. It didn't make me happy; it only made me fat.

I'll just have one. If I could have just one, why have I been fat for 20 years? I've been eating for decades, and one was never enough. Stop lying to myself. If I don't take the first little taste, if I don't begin, I won't have any problem.

One pretzel won't hurt. I've gained more weight with my fingers than with my mouth. Remember, I'm a chain eater with finger foods.

Those rolls look so good. Stop looking at and glorifying the very food that makes me fat. What am I looking at? I know what rolls look like – I'm wearing 10 pounds of them now. It's not free; I have to wear it.

Those desserts must taste good. Thin tastes better.

I'll feel deprived if I don't have a dessert. The only real deprivation *thinking* as well as their weight. Changing your thinking is necessary to change your behaviour. One technique I've developed for this was the subject of my keynote address at the National Weight Control and Obesity Symposium a number of years ago. It's called cognitive switching.

You can actually switch your thinking about how you eat by talking to yourself in a new way, then reinforcing it. The cognitive switch of the winners replaces the old, defeatist way of thinking about food that only tempts you to overeat with a new way that matches your goals. (See 'What the Winners Say' below for examples of cognitive switching.)

Strategy No. 9: Think substitution, not deprivation. The mark of what I call 'great substitute' foods is that they are light, delicious alternatives to higher-calorie foods. They have a similar look and texture as their higher-calorie counterparts, and they must taste

is never being thin. I've already spent 10 years being fat due to eating desserts. I'm living my life backward. I'm putting a piece of food before my body and my right to be thin and healthy. Was I in paradise when I was eating desserts? No! I was fat and miserable.

I blew it by eating the french fries, so I stopped trying and ate everything. I was very bad! I didn't blow it; I had a break in control. Everyone makes mistakes when learning a new skill. I contain the mistakes and move forward.

Every time I see sweets, I crave them. A craving is a feeling – not a command. Feelings pass. There'll be no pain, no blood loss. I will not have to call the emergency services. Studies show that cravings pass in minutes. If I don't negotiate or equivocate, isn't thin worth a few minutes?

I bought it for company, but I ate most of it. Thin starts in the supermarket! If I don't buy it, I don't have to wear it. I'm the easiest client to help; I've gained all my weight in my own kitchen. If I control what I put in that one room, I control my weight.

great too, so they leave you satisfied. They literally give you the taste without the calories. Most of the foods are relatively new to the market and I'll discuss them in a little more detail in the diet chapter – but right now, here are some examples of how these foods can be helpful.

For a chocolate dessert, have one of the new breed of very low-cal chocolate mousses. Flood a craving for something sweet with liquids such as diet hot chocolate (good for PMS) or a flavoured low-cal shake.

Drown a salty craving with a Tomato Cup-a-Soup or a V8 tomato juice. For salty/crunchy cravings – pickles are excellent!

Most of my clients say that substituting such foods has made all the difference in wiping out cravings and feelings of deprivation.

Strategy No. 10: Mental rehearsal. The *mental rehearsal* technique is a powerful preventive strategy when going into a situation with food you know is a major stumbling block for you. I developed this technique exclusively for my clients, and with it, you can actually desensitize yourself *in advance* to the power of that food to tempt you.

My studies in the psychology of learning taught me that the human psyche gets bored quickly with constant repetition. *Mental rehearsal* uses this trick to turn us off to the very foods that tempt us the most.

First, identify what foods you will find the most tempting in terms of sight and smell in the situation you are preparing for. Then repeat to yourself something like this: *I will smell pizza when I walk through the door, or I will smell cookies baking. Or I will see the desserts.* And then tell yourself: *It doesn't work for me. And I don't want to wear it! This is the food that made me fat.* Then put a negative association with the food – your highest weight, a part of your body where you can't stand the fat. Imagine the food going to your thighs, your bottom, or a bloated face the next day. Imagine the bulging stomach such foods have given you.

Keep repeating it till you get bored with the repetition and you say to yourself, *Enough already!* The whole thing takes just 1 to 3 minutes. Most of my clients can do it in a minute. What it does is reprogramme your mind against the two strongest elements of cravings: seeing and smelling. So when you walk into the situation, the food won't have that magnetic pull on you any longer. All of us who have gone into a beautiful restaurant or party know what it's like to look at something and think, *Wow, that looks interesting.* Mental rehearsal takes away that 'wow effect'. The few minutes it takes can save you thousands of calories and endless days and hours in the gym!

We all have power over the feeling of deprivation –
the ability to control it, decrease it, even extinguish it –
because the source of it begins and ends within you.

The Eighth Thin Commandment:
Stop Feeling Deprived

COMMANDMENT ESSENTIALS

- Change your mindset – not just your eating habits.
- Learn to Thinspeak (supporting yourself with motivational, not demoralizing, words).
- Reward yourself with a new outfit or piece of jewellery instead of food.
- Let your old trigger foods go, and embrace the delicious foods that won't put you at war with yourself.
- Remember, thin tastes better.
- Record and then regularly listen to an empowerment tape to help you think and feel like a weight-control winner.

DO YOU RECOGNIZE YOURSELF in this scenario? You've been dieting for several weeks. Your clothes are getting looser. You're seeing more definition in your face. You have more stamina. You're getting compliments about how great you look and how much weight you've lost. And then, you start getting sloppy. You begin snacking again at night, dipping into nuts or crisps or sweets, or you return to skipping meals. You've worked so hard, you're approaching your goal, you're almost there…and then you sabotage yourself, and the weight starts rolling back, or your weight loss comes to a crashing halt as you create a plateau with the extra calories. For others, the backslide may come a little later, when they are on maintenance.

This point in the weight–control process – the threshold of achievement – is one of the most critical spots you'll encounter when losing weight or trying to keep it off, a place where you're most likely to relapse into old eating habits. Call it 'diet burnout' or whatever you want, but at this point, with success at hand, many people find themselves saying, 'I don't feel like doing this anymore. I'm missing out on the fun. It's not fair. Everybody else is eating it.'

Sound familiar? Take a look at your own food history. How many times before have you returned to the foods, places or behaviours that torpedoed your efforts at weight loss right out of the water? And how often was it because you felt that you were being deprived of your favourite goodies and treats, and you felt you wanted to eat 'normally'?

Frequently, with my clients, I point out that this is the only area of their lives where they've never learned to live with success. Just as they begin to taste victory, they return to old behaviours. 'What's wrong with me? Why do I keep doing this again and again?' they often ask.

IS THIN WORTH 5 MILLION DOLLARS?

Rose, a financial executive, came to see me after many years of successfully losing weight and then, invariably, regaining it. She was just turning 40, and she didn't want to start another decade of her life repeating the same pattern of yo-yo dieting. For the past 20 years, every morning she'd awoken thinking about her weight, dreading the moment when she had to face her wardrobe and decide what she would wear for the day. Rose didn't even keep any full–length mirrors in her home. She found it depressing to see her own reflection.

'I'm not as rich as some of the people I work with on Wall Street,' she told me at our first session, 'but through the deals I've brokered, I've managed to save about 5 million dollars – and I'd gladly give it all away to end this struggle in my life. I feel confident that I know how to make more money, but I don't know how I can lose my weight and keep it off.'

Part of the reason that accomplished and successful women like Rose and so many others falter and return to self-defeating eating patterns is because, although they've lost the weight many times, they've never changed their thinking. Dieting is a pain-motivated goal. We go on diets because we're unhappy, but as soon as we drop a few pounds or kilos, we become happier and motivation fades. But that's only half the story. We might all rally a little more motivation and commitment, and we might stick with our diets till the end if only – if only we didn't feel we were missing something.

This sense of deprivation is the mindset behind the behaviours – it's the self-talk that generates the actions. It often flies under the radar, eluding our awareness completely, but it's the greater problem. This is the underlying thinking that says any guidelines are *bad* – you should be able to eat it all and *still* be thin. This way of thinking is akin to a child who has to have everything he sees and doesn't care about the consequences.

Dieting has always been associated with deprivation. The two words resonate together like flip sides of the same coin. Yet in 2005, that's old thinking. A central goal of this book is to prove to you, through the foods and 'five-star recipes' that I've given in the food chapter, that dieting is no longer about deprivation, but about substitution. In my 10-day TurboCharge Diet (see page 219), I will show you how to enjoy gourmet meals while still losing weight. Today, with many restaurants serving salads and light main course selections, dining out shouldn't be a problem either. My clients don't complain that they can't lead lives of normal eating. On the contrary, they're surprised at just how easy it is to make the transition to a diet that includes delicious foods and gives creative strategies for dining at restaurants and parties.

Although changes in food culture have been taking place, and some great products have been coming into the marketplace over the past 3 or 4 years, the programming and the mindset about deprivation has been in place in the human psyche for many years, even decades, and it won't be easily displaced without a conscious effort. Other diet programmes don't deal with it. They don't discuss managing feelings of deprivation or suggest strategies to prevent them. However, my clients and I have spent a large percentage of our time together examining this phenomenon over the years. Our conclusion? *Overcoming the deprivation mindset is a key and critical dynamic for success at weight control.*

Deprivation is triggered by behaviours, thinking and, on occasion, failing to act. Sometimes, we even think and behave in ways that fuel it. Mastering deprivation means changing both your thinking and your behaviour. It also means learning the techniques and skills that will help you defuse and even defeat the deprivation mindset. In this chapter, I'll take you through the steps and show you how to…

1. Change the mindset that's generating the behaviours

2. Use strategies to minimize or prevent feelings of deprivation

3. Deal with deprivation issues head-on

4. Go beyond deprivation to liberation

THE DEEDS THAT DEFEAT YOU

Before you bought this book and started learning about this programme, you had all of the foods you wanted, whenever you wanted them, but that freedom didn't make you happy — it only made you heavy! If you're like most people, the truth is, the more you eat, the worse you feel. And chances are that you bought this book to be rescued from the foods that have made you heavy again and again. Nevertheless, you most likely still fear the idea of being separated from the pleasure of dining — the whole concept of dieting is still imprinted on your psyche as deprivation.

Why is it so easy to feel deprived? Because people want immediacy — now! Although the goals for weight loss are long-term, they are actually pretty short-lived on the scale of life's problems. Most people on a diet can start to see noticeable changes in 10 to 30 days. After 90 days, the results will show dramatically. You don't have to get to the final goal to start seeing a payoff. The moment you experience the first signs of improvement, you're at a turning point in the process of weight loss — and this stage is easily undermined and overwhelmed by the deprivation mindset. To start wavering is human.

When temptations and cravings come into the picture, it's a high-risk, full-alert food situation for anyone who is trying to watch her weight. Giving in, giving yourself the 'gift' of this 'treat' feels normal. Denying it to yourself makes you feel deprived. Some individuals even suffer from what I call the 'Eve Complex', the tendency to feel an even greater desire for something that is restricted or forbidden, just as Eve had everything but couldn't resist the forbidden fruit in the Garden of Eden.

Don't blame yourself for responding this way. It's basic: when something gives us pleasure, we want to return to it again and again. In this way, we're no different from any creature in the animal kingdom. This is the pleasure principle that pushes human behaviour on the most fundamental level. But we do have one advantage – an intervening variable – the ability to be aware of the cost and consequences of our choices.

Of course, your favourite foods taste good, and they're delicious; that's why you love them – until a few minutes after they're down the hatch.

By definition, it's almost impossible for most middle-class people to be truly *deprived* of food. Indeed, the opposite is true; we are drowning in an overabundance of food. Recent World Health Organization statistics indicated that for the first time in human history, the number of people who are overweight exceeds the number of people who are underfed or starving. Children living in poverty are deprived. Families trapped in war-torn cities are deprived. Prisoners on starvation rations are deprived. But the fact is, if you have an interest or need to read this book, I'm fairly certain that you can eat anything you want, anytime you want. The ultimate decision to eat or not to eat is always yours.

Objectively, the state of deprivation may be a myth, but the feeling is very real. What many people don't realize is that it's also a learned response. And what has been learned can be unlearned. *We all have power over the feeling of deprivation. You have the ability to control it, decrease it, even extinguish it, because the source of it begins and ends within you.*

By becoming aware and zeroing in on your own thinking and behaviour, you can eliminate the causes and the processes that ignite deprivation. You may not realize it, but your thoughts trigger your deprivation, which in turn triggers your behaviour. Change your thoughts, learn a new response, practise it until it becomes automatic, and you will, at last, stop fuelling your own deprivation. You'll cut it off, nip it in the bud, release yourself from the prison of being controlled by food and be free to get on with the business of getting – and living – trim. The winners who have come to this realization no longer feel deprived, but liberated.

THE THOUGHTS THAT MISLEAD YOU

The diet advice that abounds on every bookstore shelf and in magazines doesn't discuss the deprivation mindset because most professionals in the field aren't trained to address changing thinking and feeling. But with my background in psychology and my study of the motivational techniques of the advertising world, I've been heavily influenced about how to change thinking – and how to replace nonproductive behaviours with behaviours that are productive.

This is the essence of good therapy of all kinds, including weight therapy, and any weight programme that doesn't deal with an individual's underlying mental and emotional orientations will be inadequate. Since most diet plans are exclusively about the right foods, right calories and right carbohydrates, it's clear why we have such a high rate of failure. Most programmes are doomed because they omit the principal motivators and determinants of successful human behaviour. As I have said before, diets are just words on a page – acting and succeeding on them is all about the right behaviour and the right motivation.

Changing the feelings of deprivation is beyond the scope of the current thinking in the field, but for me and my clients, it's at the core of our efforts. We work intensely together to make the critical shift in thinking.

It's not enough just to change your habits, your mindset has to change too.

Throughout this book, one of my core messages is about the need to abandon childhood food thinking. Here, again, it's important to understand that adult behaviour is about making choices. As we grow older, we have a restricted calorie budget. We have to make smart food choices, and over time, it becomes harder to distinguish our food choices from our life choices. Breaking with the psychology of dieting and its association with deprivation is a profound growth step.

Only children think they can have it all. And if they don't, they are therefore deprived. Yet this is the same thinking that envelops the weight-loss industry. This is what we are being led to believe. As I've explained before, some leading diet experts are the chief reinforcers of the myth that if you're denied something, you'll binge. By now it

(continued on page 150)

9 Behaviours That Increase a Feeling of Deprivation

In a survey of my clients, here are the actions that they find the most important to avoid – and, when counteracted, some of the best ways to ensure success.

1. **Allowing too much proximity.** Keeping all the foods that tempt you around and on display at home fuels a sense of deprivation. Even if you don't eat it, being near a favourite food, just knowing it's in the next room, creates a mental tug-of-war. It's always on your mind, particularly if it's clearly visible. In public settings, 'no proximity' means try not to sit near or make eye contact with foods that tempt you. *Control your food curiosity.* Don't go grazing in 'food temples' such as supermarkets or delicatessens, don't read the sections of a menu with foods you are trying to avoid, and don't survey the dessert menu, hors d'oeuvres or other foods that tempt you. Remember that the more you centre your life on a vulnerability, the more vulnerable your life will become! Availability stimulates craving – it's that simple!

2. **Telling yourself that if you can't have it, you'll be deprived.** Behind this statement is the assumption that *it's not normal; everyone else is having it.* But over the years, everyone who's said this to me has overlooked one obvious truth: their weight has never been normal because of the foods they're so worried about missing out on. I tell them to worry more about a normal weight, a normal life, normal health and normal sizes than what everyone else is eating.

3. **Going too long without eating.** If you're starving, just seeing and smelling food will have a powerful impact.

4. **Going into food situations unprepared.** A simple truth of behaviour is that if people don't have the right foods around them, eventually they'll eat the wrong ones. If you go into a conference room meeting for a day, and pastries or biscuits or other foods that are a problem for you are being served, and you haven't brought your ThinPack of low-calorie snacks along, you will eat what is there, or you will feel a constant struggle with temptation.

5. **Forgetting that you know what it tastes like.** You've already tasted it all; there are no more surprises. You know the taste and texture of virtually every food imaginable – what more can it give you?

6. **Tasting trigger foods that you've decided to Box Out.** Don't forget that you can't have 'just a little' of the foods that have been a problem for you historically. As I've said many times before, taking a taste of a trigger food may reactivate your cravings and unleash your thinking, looking and obsessing about it. Invariably, tasting foods that you have decided to Box Out makes it harder, because the pleasure principle of the human psyche makes you want to finish it and have more and not be a 'taster'. It's not about the calories in a taste but about the cravings and food interest that taste reactivates.

7. **Not giving yourself alternative rewards.** You can minimize your deprivation response before entering a risky food situation by doing a Mental Rehearsal and reminding yourself of your new reward system – both are very effective uses of psychology. Tell yourself that you won't eat the french fries, but you'll buy yourself a beautiful outfit or you'll do something you love. This technique is a favourite among my clients.

8. **Failing to embrace the substitutes.** In today's food culture, the choices for low-calorie, low-fat foods are so wide, there are enough to accommodate every personal taste and preference. Studies show that if you don't have your favourite food, but you have your second favourite, you're better able to control it. For example, my clients who love chocolate cookies find that chocolate mousse is very satisfying, but without the crunch that would trigger compulsive overeating.

9. **Forgetting that eating a food is not free.** Once you realize the high cost of a behaviour, it reduces the attractiveness of that behaviour – meaning that eating a food that sabotages your weight loss or your control is not a 'treat' but a costly decision. Don't confuse a 'great taste' with a 'great life'. The major reason you have been miserable or unhappy with your weight is because of these types of foods. See yourself at your highest weight and ask yourself the powerful question that breaks any feeling of deprivation: 'Do I like it enough to wear it?' When you realize the fact that you may already be wearing several pounds of this food, ask yourself, 'Do I really need another serving of such a "treat"?'

should be no big surprise to see me write again that when it comes to trigger foods, once you stop eating them and keeping them around, you lose a great deal – if not all – of your cravings. And most people find that they don't miss them once they realize the true cost of eating them. Although it may be difficult at first to let go of trigger foods, the long-term benefits far outweigh any short-term discomforts. My clients and I have found that it is easier to say 'no' than to just have a little.

Sample Tape No. 2: Keeping the Winners' Edge

To begin your tape, name the specific foods that have caused you to feel deprived. Think about what has happened to your weight when these foods are in your life. Then proceed with the rest of the dialogue.

- 'Today, I will stay focused on what is essential, and I will not waste my time on what is nonessential. I will have flipped the switch that turns off the thoughts of deprivation in my head. I've seen it all and tasted it all in the world of food. I can succeed at being trim. Each time I say, "No, thank you," I say, "yes" to being trim and successful. Only the thin say, "No, thank you." To be in control is empowering. To have the power to say, "No, thank you," to that which has destroyed my figure (or control) again and again is

liberating. I don't need to look at it, think about it or taste it. I've had enough for three lifetimes.'

- Emphasize why you had your weight problem. 'Yes, this food (name it) has a pleasant taste for a few moments, but these few moments have cost me years, decades of misery. It's just a piece of food. Don't be a "food whiner" and make yourself miserable. You can have all you want, whenever you want, but you'll never have the life you want.'

- 'By taking it one day at a time, I'm building a lifetime of being in control. If I find myself obsessing about a piece of food, I will tell myself, "Get over it; you're already wearing it. If it made you so happy, why were you always so miserable about your weight?"'

- 'I will remember all that I want to

A Tale of Two Wardrobes

My client, Martha, had lost weight and regained it so often that she had several sets of clothing, one in her favourite size, the others in increasingly larger sizes. Fortunately, she had two wardrobes in her bedroom. She kept her preferred clothes in one and her collection of larger sizes in the other. One morning, she opened the wrong wardrobe by mistake. That day, she needed to dress in one of her larger outfits, since her weight had been creeping up for several weeks. But when she opened the wrong wardrobe and caught a

do, and I won't worry about any foods that may divert me. I don't live in a fairyland where I can have it all and still be trim, but that doesn't mean I'm deprived. I have so much going for me; I deserve to be in control. I deserve to be trim. I deserve to succeed in the world of food. I won't let my PMS, or the Poor Me Syndrome, block my memory and make me forget that when I had it all, I ate it all and I was miserable. Being in control with my weight and my food makes me feel empowered each day, makes me feel better about myself and makes me look better. Complacency is the enemy of thin. Letting myself get sloppy because of the compliments I'm getting is to not understand that every time people say to me how great I look, how much weight I lost, they're also thinking how fat I was before. If I let the compliments go to my head, they'll soon grow silent again as I regain the weight.'

- 'Every so often, I may just see or smell a food that tempts me. I'll say to myself, "It's just for the moment," because I'm just seeing/smelling it. It's just a feeling, not a command. Feelings pass, but the taste of trim can endure for a lifetime when I say, "No thanks," to this food(s). It doesn't work for me, that's why...I don't begin; I don't have any problem!'

- 'In eating this way, I will look years younger. I will feel more attractive and more empowered. There are setbacks in life, and although being thin doesn't guarantee I'll be happy, it does guarantee that I won't be unhappy because I'm fat.'

glimpse of all the stylish clothes that she would much rather be wearing and could not, she slammed the door immediately – hard.

'It was at that moment,' she told me later, 'I realized that the true deprivation came *from* eating all of the foods that had caused my weight to balloon. My behaviour had *deprived me* of wearing the clothes I loved.'

The insight that had hit Martha, which she helped me to see when she shared her story, is that we experience liberation only when we are free to live as we choose, not as hostages to a piece of food, taking orders from cravings and suffering from a gnawing feeling that we're missing out on something.

Today, both of Martha's wardrobes hold clothing in the same ideal size. When she thinks back to her former 'fat closet', she thinks: 'Never again.' She enjoys wearing her beautiful clothes and looking her best, and she knows she'll always have the strategies to keep her in control – and liberated!

BACK TALK THAT WORKS

Deprivation doesn't just happen; it's something that is done to you. The feelings that you've experienced on previous diets, of missing out on something, were produced by the programming of your past, the pre-recorded mindset, which you, in turn, perpetuate and impose on yourself. Whenever you are near food, the old tape switches on and these messages go to work fostering your feelings of deprivation and eroding your control over food.

Most of my clients find it easy to see the effects of this programming when they are in my office. They realize that foods that consistently trigger overeating or endless cravings are enemies, not treats. They know that the real deprivation is in never living trim. But self-talk isn't always conscious or even rational. It was 'taped' long ago and reinforced ever since. As a result, even the most logical and determined dieters can find themselves thinking, 'I can't live without it', when they know perfectly well there is nothing essential to survival in a chocolate bar or a potato crisp.

It will make me feel better. It will make me happy. It will comfort me. This thinking is at the core of the deprivation mindset, and the greatest thing you can do is to eclipse these thoughts and connect to a new voice. A food that you enjoy for comfort shouldn't bring you discomfort.

Learning to rewrite your internal dialogue can be the difference between success and failure. It can speed you along the road away from the deprivation mindset, or it can drag you back and keep you enslaved to your trigger foods. The choice is yours, because with time and practice, you can erase your old self-talk and replace it with positive, realistic messages. Those who succeed at weight control engage in a supportive inner dialogue. Simply put, their words to themselves are motivating, not demoralizing, and when they're faced with old programming, they dare to talk back. So can you. Here are a few sample retorts to get you started.

LEARNING TO THINSPEAK

I'm missing out on the fun.	What fun? You had it for years and it didn't make you happy – it only made you fat.
Everybody's eating it.	True or not, you've had enough for three lifetimes.
What's wrong with a taste?	Taking a taste makes it harder. (Most people can taste most foods, but as I've discussed at length, some individuals have a long history of abusing a single food or type of food. In these cases, it's easier to rule out the food entirely. Taking a taste is like an ex-smoker taking a cigarette. It's restarting the pattern. It's better not to think about it at all, much like getting over a failed love affair. Take a taste only if your history indicates you have been a 'taster' with this food; otherwise, avoid it.)
I just want it.	I want to be thin even more. I don't want it enough to wear it.
It's so hard.	Being fat is harder.

If you don't do the strategies, if you go too long without eating and if you don't eat low-calorie substitutes, it *will* seem hard. If you think you can't or that you have to give up the pleasure of fine food for a lifetime, it will seem *impossibly* hard. But hopefully, all the lessons in this book have already convinced you that being thin isn't about giving up the fun in your life or the pleasure of great dining – it's about giving up sloppy compulsive eating behaviours and habits that keep you from succeeding.

Turning Off the Deprivation Switch

Deprivation is a learned experience – most of the people on earth have never seen or tasted the majority of the foods that many of us 'can't live without'. It's a learned cultural experience. *And what can be learned can be unlearned* is a central theme of this book.

One of the most efficient ways to deprogramme yourself is to make a tape. When you're feeling deprived, the mechanism busily at work within you is the voice in your head. In a way, you're sub-jecting yourself to self-hypnosis: 'I have to have it. I have to have it. If I don't, I'm deprived.'

It's one thing to understand this intellectually, but it's dramati-cally more effective to enhance what you know through the power of listening to a tape or CD, which will instil a new message into your subconscious – and you actually feel it!

Use this tool to turn off the feelings of deprivation. Counteract them. Give yourself a new internal dialogue.

There are two major reasons why my clients don't find the work we do together hard. One is strategy. The other is that they don't feel deprived. You can have the same benefits by making a tape for yourself. It's not required, but it will make it easier to defeat the deprivation mindset. If you choose not to tape, you can get some of the same effects by writing key statements from the sample script on Post-its and putting them up around your home. Being a winner is a matter of thinking and feeling like a winner. You can get all the lessons simply from reading this book, but you can get them more quickly and effectively if you make yourself a tape. Realize that you're listening to a tape already, every day, running through your head. This strategy just sub-stitutes a new tape full of empowering visions for you and your life so that you can think like a winner.

You can eat like a millionaire in the world of calories and still look like a million.

The Ninth Thin Commandment:
Treat Your Calories Like Money

COMMANDMENT ESSENTIALS

- Eat high-calcium dairy foods and cinnamon, both of which make fat cells behave more efficiently.
- Substitute delicious light versions of your favourite foods for calorie-laden 'fat' versions.
- Drink plenty of water to help keep calories and carbs from being stored as fat.
- Watch for hidden calories, such as the right foods being prepared the wrong way.
- Spend your calories only on foods you really care about.
- Eat foods that provide high satiety, but low calories.

YOU'RE IN THE SUPERMARKET BUYING FOIL. Two brands of similar quality have the same price, but one reads: '30 per cent more free!' Which one would you choose?

So would I.

We deeply respect our money and with good reason. We work hard and only have so much. No one needs to be told: 'Get the most for your money.'

We also need to respect our *calories*. Your body works hard to burn them, and when you overspend, you end up wearing them. Indeed, for most of us, calories cost more than money: in larger-size clothes, discomfort, depression and reduced life expectancy. The good news is that you already have the know-how to profit from your calories: you can *approach weight control simply as an accounting issue. Treat your calories like money, and get the most for your pound or dollar!*

CALORIENOMICS: STRETCHING YOUR CALORIE BUDGET

Calorienomics is the strategy of treating your calories like money. *You want to get greater value for less cost.* The goal of calorienomics is to be able to eat more food while lessening the calories but not the pleasure of eating – and still lose weight! How's that for a diet plan you can live with?

One of the comments I hear from my clients again and again is that they're eating much more than they were before – and more frequently! And they wonder, especially at the start, if they'll ever lose weight this way.

You wouldn't be reading this book if they didn't.

The secret is that they're also eating more *wisely* – according to the principles of calorienomics. And many also say they're eating with as much or *greater* enjoyment than they did with the foods that made them gain weight.

Just as salary or income determines a budget, certain factors contribute to your body's calorie budget. While genetics sets the lower limit for our weight, *we* set the upper limit by how we spend our calories. Genetics, food choices and how much you move – these factors give your body *a fixed budget.* It varies from person to person, but *each of us has a given number of calories to spend.* And if you're reading this book, you're having trouble living within your calorie budget, and you want to know the best way to readjust your spending. But – just as with your economic budget – you don't want to sacrifice needlessly or do without the things you care about most.

All of us would like to have it all – but it isn't possible. It would be great to walk into any shop and buy whatever we want, but that's not a realistic scenario. Who can walk into their favourite clothes shop and spend a whole month's salary on an outfit when the rent or mortgage is due?

But often the people who buy so thoughtfully will nibble mindlessly on whatever's in front of them or blow almost a week's weight loss on a bowl of cashews. The same meticulous people who pore over bank statements for unnecessary costs don't think to wonder what outrageous calories lie hidden in a salad dressing or restaurant sauce. The same ones who buy 'value packs' or comparison-shop don't realize what calorie bargains there are in the world of delicious foods. These behaviours give new meaning to that old English saying: 'Penny-wise, pound-foolish'!

We don't want to be like the child in the toy shop having a tantrum because he can't have all he sees, feeling deprived and missing out on all the goodies. Calorienomics uses your adult budgeting skills and common sense to stretch your calorie budget in ways that allow you to have the *foods* as well as the figure you love.

Four principles guide calorienomics:

1. Finding foods that are low in calories but high in taste, nutrition and satiety (how full they make you feel).

2. Finding foods the body uses in a way that promotes greater loss of weight than other foods with equal calories. These 'body-friendly' foods either kill appetite with small amounts or give you few calories with large amounts.

3. Finding the very best light substitutes for your favourite foods, those that are closest in taste, texture, look and satisfaction to the originals. They keep the taste without the calories.

4. Avoiding the foods and *behaviours* that bust your budget and participating in behaviours that *stretch* it.

The goal of calorienomics is to give you the freedom to *eat more and lose more*. Many diets like to promise that, but calorienomics shows you how to *do* it – easily and simply. Like a good budget that enables a well-rounded life, calorienomics respects the biological *and* social role of food in our lives as well as the need of the psyche for volume, rich taste and texture. The diet plan you'll find in our food chapter (see page 196) was designed to meet these very goals:

delicious meals and snacks that give you great taste and volume with less calories, that make the body burn calories more efficiently and that end hunger and cravings. Our calorienomic food plan also helps you painlessly save up calories for those special foods you love as well as the special celebrations you enjoy over food.

Like all of the other commandments in this book, calorienomics provides you with a complete strategy for enjoying your life at a weight that makes you look good and feel good.

THE BUDGET STRETCHERS

You've probably heard it said, 'A calorie is a calorie.' That may be true in laboratory research, where a calorie is a unit for measuring heat. But in looking at how calories affect weight loss and appetite, some calories are clearly 'more equal than others'. *Some calories work more efficiently than others in lowering weight or controlling appetite.*

It takes calories to burn calories, and some require more burning than others to get digested and absorbed. And some calories quench appetite, whereas others stimulate it. There are also calories that control appetite and cravings by keeping insulin levels stable. By choosing your calories wisely, you can optimize the body's processes for weight loss without losing taste or volume. These budget stretchers biologically frustrate fat while meeting your psychological needs for satiety and the pleasure of foods you enjoy.

Budget Stretcher No. 1: The Thermogenic Effect of Food. Food gives calories, but also takes them away. Digestion requires energy and calories are what the body burns for energy. The amount of caloric energy it takes to break down any given food is called its *thermogenic effect*. This effect accounts for 5 to 10 per cent of your metabolic rate, which can make a critical difference in boosting weight loss and maintaining it.

Lean protein has the most thermogenic effect of all foods. It is estimated to use up roughly 30 per cent of its calories for digestion. Simple carbohydrates such as baked goods, pastries or regular white pasta have poor thermogenic effects, burning around 6 to 8 per cent of their calories in thermogenesis. Fat calories are the lowest, burning about 3 per cent of their calories before going straight to storage (usually on your hips!).

The four thermogenic winners that really exercise your metabolism and work hardest to end your appetite are: white-meat fish and seafood, vegetables that are high-fibre and low-starch, egg whites and fibre.

But you can eat more of the thermogenic foods that are lower in calories per ounce than the high-carb grains. An egg white omelette, for example, with spinach and mushrooms gives you a complete meal for about the calories of half a cup of brown rice. And I have clients who snack on a pound of green beans every day, and they still lose weight. But I don't think they'd have the same success with a pound of wholegrain pasta or brown rice. While whole grains are certainly nutritious, people often have problems with their quantities. This poses a behavioural problem for weight-control success, particularly when a serving of cooked pasta, rice, or other grains amounts to about the size of a tennis ball, and most people will eat much more than that amount in the real world.

The perfect solution to getting the benefit of grain without the danger of volume is the unique GG Scandinavian Bran Crispbread I describe earlier in this book and in the food chapter (see page 204). For a fraction of the calories, it gives you as much fibre as the best grains plus large volume. Great crunch…and for you carb watchers, zero net carbs per serving – find a pasta, rice or even another cracker that can do that!

Budget Stretcher No. 2: Foods That Make Fat Cells Behave More Efficiently. Imagine the bonus of a food that comes in wide variety, has great taste, promotes weight loss, kills appetite and burns fat instead of storing it! In studies that give the same amount of calories to two groups of dieters, the group that gets this food *loses 70 per cent more weight* than the group that doesn't. The research shows that this product particularly is good for a trim waistline and a flat stomach. Plus, it's available in every supermarket! What's this '70 per cent-edge food?' High-calcium dairy foods.

And there's also a food with *zero* calories that helps weight loss, kills your appetite and stabilizes your blood sugar with less than a teaspoon of it per day. This food is a delicious spice – cinnamon.

We discuss both these foods – as well as how to use them creatively to promote weight loss *and* great dining – in the food chapter.

Budget Stretcher No. 3: Substitution. Let's face it, in the real world, many of the foods we love are high in calories.

Indeed, many of the foods that are *worst* for us and our weight control have a great taste. We want to lose weight, but not the pleasure of that taste.

Food manufacturers have received much blame for the obesity problem, but now they are becoming part of the *solution*. Their intense research into what foods people crave the most are resulting in delicious light versions. They are cutting calories, carbs and fat in everything from dressings and snack foods to delicious chocolate mousses. These days, even fast-food chains are coming to our rescue, with many offering tasty, light-calorie substitutes for high-cal fattening meals.

Budget Stretcher No. 4: Satiety. Certain foods fill you up quickly, so you don't have to eat very much, yet you're not hungry. In a recent satiety study, of all the foods tested, which two stood alone at the top of the list? Fish was right up there with the boiled potato! Beating the grains, the breads – even oatmeal.

Budget Stretcher No. 5: Can a Fruit Help You Lose Extra Weight? For years, supporters of grapefruit diets have contended that eating that citrus fruit was a surefire way to lose weight.

Now, new research has confirmed their claim. A study at one of America's leading hospitals, the Scripps Clinic's Nutrition and Metabolic Research Center, has revealed that people eating three servings of grapefruit a day with their meals lost 1.4–2.25 kg (3–5 lb) a month *without changing their existing diet*. Many patients lost more than 4.5 kg (10 lb).

The study participants consumed three servings of grapefruit a day, in the form of either 240 ml (8 fl oz) of grapefruit juice, half a grapefruit, or special capsules of freeze-dried grapefruit with meals. The group that ate the fresh grapefruit lost an average of 1.6 kg (3.6 lb) in 30 days, the juice drinkers lost 1.5 kg (3.3 lb), and the participants who took the capsules lost 1.1 kg (2.4 lb).

The researchers conjecture that the chemical properties of grapefruit reduce insulin levels and promote weight loss. The importance of this link may have to do with the hormone's function in weight management. While weight management is not its primary function, insulin assists with the regulation of fat metabolism. So the smaller the insulin spike after a meal, the more efficiently the body processes food for use as energy and the less calories are stored as fat in the body. Grapefruit may possess unique chemical properties that reduce the insulin levels that encourage weight loss.

Dr Ken Fujioka, principal researcher at the Nutrition and Metabolic Research Center, said, 'Whether it's the properties of grapefruit or its ability to satiate appetites, grapefruit appeared to help with weight loss and decreased insulin levels, leading to better health.'

What is most significant about the study is that the patients lost the weight without otherwise changing their diet. This debunks the longstanding axiom that a calorie is just a calorie, and all calories are the same. Obviously, the calories of some foods work better than others for weight loss purposes, and this study suggests that grapefruit should be added to the list of calorie stretchers.

I am just beginning to test this 'budget stretcher' in my own practice but I wanted to share this late-breaking new research with you.

(*Note:* Individuals taking heart medication should not consume grapefruit with their medication. Please check with your doctor on how many hours should elapse between taking your heart medication and eating grapefruit.)

Budget Stretcher No. 6: Water – The Magic Elixir. The effects of water on weight may not be fully understood or appreciated as of 2005, but it has always been my observation that *water promotes weight loss.*

Most dieters don't drink enough water. To metabolize 1 gram of carbohydrate, for example, your body needs 3 grams of fluid. So drinking enough water can help keep your carbs from being stored as fat. One study suggests that water suppresses appetite, but it's better to drink before a meal than wash your food through your body with large amounts during the meal. Another very recent study shows that after two glasses of water, your system 'shifts into high gear and starts burning fat'. And German researchers found that people who consume two 240-ml (8-fl oz) glasses of water increased their rate of calorie burning by 30 per cent about 40 minutes later, and it stayed elevated for more than an hour. Think strategy and drink the water 40 to 60 minutes before a meal so you'll have the calories of the meal more efficiently metabolized. The researchers estimate that drinking eight 240-ml (8-fl oz) glasses of water a day –

the minimum recommended amount – could burn off an extra 35,000 calories a year, or 4.5 kg (10 lb). There is also evidence that reasonable amounts of *cold* water make your metabolism burn calories to warm you back up (because cold water lowers your body temperature). Elington Darden, PhD, author of *Living Longer Stronger*, says 'Drinking more ice cold water causes more heat transfer throughout the skin,' which indicates calorie-burning. (He goes on to say that even 'staying cool instead of being hot will facilitate fat loss two and three times over and above the normal rate'.)

Proper hydration helps you with your weight programme in other ways. When you begin a diet, your body loses fluid as well as weight. Without adequate fluid, you're more prone to water retention and constipation, which can keep your scales from accurately reflecting your weight loss. In addition, dehydration can make you feel weak or headachy, which in turn can make you want to move and exercise less as well as eat more for additional energy. When dehydrated, all your body systems slow down, so it's good to monitor your body's hydration. Use what I call 'the colour test': make sure your urine is white to straw-coloured by midday. Then you'll know your body has adequate fluid to conduct its normal calorie-burning processes.

The exact role of water in promoting weight loss is not entirely clear – all the information is not yet in. Some weight specialists believe it may not be a significant factor; others believe it is. All I can share with you is that over the years, I've heard thousands of clients saying, 'When I drink more water, I lose more weight.' Just don't be excessive; six to eight glasses seems to be adequate for healthy people. Just check with your doctor if you have oedema, kidney problems or other medical conditions that affect your water intake.

Budget Stretcher No. 7: Use Fixed Meals. Research has shown that prepackaged meals (such as TV dinners) can significantly stretch your calorie budget. In one study, the dieters who had these portion-controlled meals lost 30 per cent more weight than the others. The reason? With fixed meals, you know exactly how many calories you're getting. Apparently, our tendency to underestimate calories is not to be underestimated! So go ahead, and enjoy the convenience of a fixed meal several times a week.

Budget Stretcher No. 8: The Exercise Edge. My clients often ask me how important it is to incorporate exercise into their weight-control regime. I say, 'Very.' But I remind them, exercise cannot compare to the exercise of good *judgement* with your food choices!

The biggest budget stretcher is eating the right foods, but exercise gives you a crucial edge. That edge, however, may not be what people think it is. Exercise's greatest contribution is to success at weight control – because it gives focus and structure. It encourages the right *behaviours* for dieters…not just the calorie burn.

BUDGET BUSTERS

Budget busters are either high-calorie foods with very low thermogenic effect (like those high in fat and refined carbohydrates) or eating *behaviours* that in various ways end up costing far too many calories.

Drink Tea for Weight Loss

We always have known that tea is delicious, refreshing and thirst-quenching and in some cases may help reduce the risk of cancer.

You can now add it to the list of no-calorie foods that may help promote weight loss.

A recent Taiwanese study, led by Dr Chih-Hsing Wu of the National Chang Kung University Medical College, Tainu, showed interesting results. The study of more than 1,100 people, reported in *Obesity Research*, revealed that those people who drank at least one glass of black, green or oolong tea per week for 10 years had 20 per cent less body fat and 2 per cent less abdominal fat than those who drank none. This was regardless of the amount of physical activity, food intake and other lifestyle habits.

The researchers surmise that the tea may raise the metabolic rate while lowering the absorption of sugars and fat-producing molecules. This study is the most recent that relates tea to weight loss and adds evidence to what has up till now been a mixed bag of results. Multiple studies have suggested that tea promotes weight loss, whereas a few others have questioned its role. The best way to answer the question is once again to try it in your own life.

Budget Buster No. 1: Eating Food 'Just Because It's There'. I would estimate that a good third to half of the calories my clients are consuming when they first see me are not from foods they particularly care about or would go out of their way to buy if they lived alone. Mostly they eat them because they happen to be around the house or office or right in front of them when they go out with other people. If it's in a bowl or basket within arm's reach, whatever it is, before long it's being nibbled on. I joke that their fingers have a 'wait problem'.

Snacks and other 'nibble foods' are what make many people prone to lose control of their calorie budgets. In the US, it's estimated that almost *a quarter of all the calories consumed may be spent on snacking* – for some people, even more! Crisps, nuts, biscuits, sweets, pretzels, fizzy drinks and so on – you can find them almost anywhere in easy-to-eat-from bags and containers. *Snacks are 'credit card foods' – they make it easy to spend your calories without realizing the cost.* Each bite seems like a small, innocent amount, but the bill at the end of the month can make your jaw drop.

Oversize portions of high-caloric foods are also a particular problem in many countries. The ever-growing portion size is a uniquely modern phenomenon. So is allowing our children to serve themselves whatever amount of high-calorie food they feel like heaping on their plates. This routine fosters feelings of deprivation when appropriate portions are served – an unhealthy attitude that's hard to break.

Years of observation have led me to form the E.A.T. principle – the Expanding Appetite Theorem: the appetite expands in direct proportion to the amount of food presented! *People are finishers.* People tend to finish what's on their plate. And the larger the plate, the more food we get served, so the more we eat. Even a larger *package* – the bag of crisps, the box of cereal, the bar of chocolate – makes us tend to eat more, independent of our hunger. This is just how humans behave, once again proving we are given to excess, not moderation, and we need strategy to control this tendency.

Even when people order healthy foods, they often ignore the quantity. So be alert for large portions or packages (especially of grains and other unmeasured nutritious foods).

Budget Buster No. 2: Eating High-Calorie Food Too Often or Indiscriminately. Some people prefer a great steak at a superb restaurant over a third-rate hamburger with dressing with just as many calories. Others would rather have a superb 500-calorie dessert at the weekend. It's one thing to save up enough calories to allow yourself a treat from time to time. But it's quite another to eat it every day because it's on your kitchen worktop or your favourite restaurant's menu. Sometimes cutting out excesses such as these just requires a simple change in how you prepare or acquire food. Instead of cooking lots for your children's dinner and finishing what your children don't eat, for example, just make enough, so there's no excess. Strive to save your highest-calorie items for special restaurants where you get superb quality or for the special events that give joy to your life.

Budget Buster No. 3: Activity Eating. Some people are shocked to realize how many calories they spend on *activity eating*: eating just to be doing something when bored, anxious or procrastinating; or eating associated with an activity, such as sitting in front of a TV or computer, talking on the phone or reading. Many people say the weekends are the toughest. With all the unstructured free time in the afternoon or an evening home, people can get bored and may find themselves picking constantly all day or watching more TV and getting something to chew on during every commercial break.

And don't forget an insider tip: keep the lights on bright and you'll snack less. People tend to eat more in dark environments, research has shown. Ah yes, moviegoers!

Budget Buster No. 4: The 10-Minute Problem in Restaurants. Ten minutes is a very short time, but it can cost you more calories than the entire day if you're not careful. It can even cancel out the calorie benefit of hours spent in the gym. Winners at weight control realize that *the first and last 10 minutes in restaurants can cost more than the meal.* Good strategy is often needed in the first 10 minutes to resist the lure of too much alcohol or the breadbasket (which – did you ever notice? – no one seems to miss in a Chinese or Japanese restaurant); and a salad dressing with more fat than a dessert. And in the *last* 10 minutes, there's the dessert question. What kind and what size portion does your budget allow?

So remember: the next time you want to reach for that roll or dessert menu – if you let the 10 minutes pass, it can save you hours in the gym. Your busy schedule will appreciate the effort!

Budget Buster No. 5: Hidden Calories. Are you over-spending without realizing it? Most people realize that eating the wrong foods causes overspending, and if they cut them out, they notice a weight loss. But often after a period, the weight loss slows down radically or even stops, and my clients say they've 'reached a plateau'. *'Reaching a plateau' is typically an early warning sign of over-spending.* I tell them they haven't reached a plateau, they've created one – usually by overlooking *hidden calories.*

Some calories hide in plain sight:

• **Too much of the right foods** – especially fruit, chicken, meat and grains – can lead to calories you hadn't counted on.

• **The right foods served with the wrong ones** – the 'sides' that come with a meal – can wipe out your calorie savings. An egg white omelette, say, that is served with fries. The targeted eating strategy when ordering your main course is to ask *What does it come with?* Don't be afraid of speaking up – you're the one paying good money for the meal, and your body is sharing the bill!

Other hidden calories are not so easy to detect:

• **The right foods prepared the wrong way** can bewilder dieters who often eat in restaurants and think they're ordering wisely but aren't losing weight. A classic example is calamari, which is very low in calories – except when cooked in butter or deep-fried! To avoid these hidden calories, always specify how you want your order prepared – even vegetables. Just saying one word – 'steamed' or 'poached' can save you 10 to 30 grams of fat on the vegetables alone. Steaming or poaching doesn't mean 'no taste'. If you ask them to steam the food with garlic and herbs or to poach it in wine or stock with herbs, most restaurants are happy to do so.

• **Salad dressing – a dessert on top of a salad.** Even the healthiest salad can cost an astonishing number of calories. An Italian salad with an olive-oil dressing can have as much fat as *two* quarter-pounders from McDonald's! Even though it may be 'good' monounsaturated oil, from a weight loss point of view, fat is fat and it's a weight-loss killer. Olive oil and Caesar salad dressings are the most common trip-ups – even the light versions. My clients often order a chicken Caesar thinking that the chicken breast makes it a light meal, forgetting that some Caesar salad dressings can set you back as much as 30 grams of fat and many more calories than the chicken itself. Perhaps that's why Caesar had to always wear a toga! So always ask for 'dressing on the side', and dip a fork into it instead of a spoon each time you want to add the dressing to your salad.

Budget Buster No. 6: Counting in Calories, Not Calorie Units. It may seem strange to say that counting calories busts your budget, but the truth is, many people may *count* in calories, but they *eat* in calorie *units*. It's not how many calories per serving that matters, but how many servings you typically eat. A few cashews may make up one serving, but most people don't stop with just a few. Or cereal – the average person pours into their breakfast bowl two to three times the amount given on the label as a single serving. And for someone with a history of finishing the whole bag of pretzels, the calories can end up three or more times the amount listed for a serving on the label. So it will serve you best to be honest about how many servings you really eat.

Budget Buster No. 7: Too Much Variety. As I pointed out earlier, variety increases consumption, particularly at home. The more types of food you have around (especially nibble foods), the more you'll pick and eat and have food on your mind – and the hungrier you may feel. *The more foods in your pantry, the fewer clothes in your closet!* But when your taste buds encounter the same foods again and again, they get satisfied quicker. Too much variety keeps them curious and slower to signal 'Enough'. You go from one variety to the next, and your quantities and frequencies of eating increase. Limiting the types of food you buy and eat, for dieters, can have very big results!

Budget Buster No. 8: Trigger Foods. Trigger foods overpower your appetite's shut-off switch. They tend to *stimulate* rather than satisfy cravings and appetite, particularly foods made from white flour or sugar. Crunchy, bite-size foods such as nuts and sweets are also hard to limit because you can quickly pop one after another mindlessly. When you surround yourself with such foods, you'll find that you're constantly thinking about them. 'Always on my mind' in this case can mean 'always on my behind'.

Busting the Busters: The Secret Weapon

To correct for these budget busters, remember a simple technique that will cost you about 2 or 3 minutes a day but can save you *months* of fruitless, frustrated dieting or even failure: *keep a food diary* (see page 32). Virtually all my clients who keep them find that they experience the same two results: (1) more awareness of hidden calories and therefore more weight loss, and (2) a much higher level of success in *keeping* the weight off.

TARGETED EATING: HONOURING YOUR PRIORITIES

Targeted eating is my strategy for avoiding or limiting the foods you care less about *so you can eat the foods you care more about or have them more often.*

Even if you extend your budget with calorienomic winners and exercise, your budget is still not infinite. First, you should spend it on food you need for good nutrition and energy. And the rest of your budget you can save for food you truly love (if you don't have a history of compulsively abusing it). For some, this might be a special dessert or even a holiday feast. Targeted eating gives you the freedom to enjoy these pleasures of your life. It builds up your calorie bank account. It also makes it easier to say no to high-calorie foods when you know you're saving the calories for something special you plan to enjoy soon.

So if you like to splurge on gourmet meals in a special restaurant or have a big dinner party coming up on the weekend, from Monday through Thursday eat 'light gourmet' with the recipes on pages 223–24 and 226). Or if you know that you're going to a celebration dinner soon, save up calories by eating seafood or my Dr G's World Famous Low-Calorie Courgette/Aubergine Parmigiana (see page 238) for a few nights before and after.

Build up your savings by being *selective* about what you eat. The reason most people are overweight is that they *want* much more than they *need*. The goal of targeted eating is to pick what you want the *most*, so you can have what you *truly* need – the looks, the good health, the control and the quality of life. Targeted eating also has the advantage of providing you with a safety zone in case you slip or fall from your diet.

Just as people save money for a rainy day, targeted eating puts calories in your body's savings account as a resource for special needs or treats – or if you should overeat. If you continue to balance your meals for good health and not spend too many calories on non-nutritious foods, targeted eating can put a great amount of pleasure in your diet.

BEING FOODSMART

Being foodSmart means picking foods that give you the *volume* you desire and let you eat more frequently. They provide high satiety but not high calories. This keeps your blood sugar stable and helps put an end to your cravings and hunger.

Winning at weight loss is never about losing the pleasure of food. Being foodSmart means finding great calorie bargains that offer great taste, satisfaction and large volume with fewer calories. The foods in the eating plan will help you become foodSmart.

High Volume, Low Calories

In 1994, when I wrote *Thin Tastes Better*, the advice of most weight counsellors was to cut the food you're served in half and leave half on the plate. The diet approach I designed strongly rejected this behaviour-modification approach to eating. All you have to do is go to a restaurant to realize this is not how real people behave. For most of my clients, there is no greater torture than sitting in a restaurant watching half your dinner grow cold as your friends finish theirs. And you still have to pay full price for half a meal! The 'eat half, leave half' diet was contrary to the way people behave and a breeding ground for feeling deprived. People like volume!

Years after my book came out, Barbara Rolls, PhD, published an important, groundbreaking work in *Volumetrics*, which confirmed my approach scientifically. Her pioneering studies documented that *people want foods they can eat in large volume*. They will choose a large amount of food that's their second choice over a smaller portion of their first choice. Being foodSmart respects this basic human desire and gives you the volume you want without the extra calories. Instead of a tiny steak, order a whole trout steamed with lemon juice and garlic or drizzled with a teaspoon of butter – for fewer calories! Or for dessert, instead of a forlorn sliver of chocolate cake have a delicious cappuccino with whipped cream. Or a low-cal chocolate mousse.

How to Save Thousands of Calories in 1 Month

Robb was a healthy but overweight man in his early thirties. A successful financial manager, he immediately understood the wisdom of calorienomics, and his expert budgeting skills and strategic mind made his diet programme smooth and successful. I'd like to describe his typical eating day to show how painlessly you can lose significant weight by targeted eating and being foodSmart.

The first thing Robb realized was that the New York–style bagel he ate every morning was more than 400 calories, plus a couple hundred more for his butter or cream cheese topping. He had no trouble switching to a toasted English muffin (110 calories) with an egg (80 calories) and a spray of light oil spray (virtually zero calories). On some days, he had 2 tablespoons of low-fat cream cheese without the egg and a glass of skimmed milk. And when he had time for something more elaborate, he'd often make the egg white omelette from my gourmet recipes.

His usual lunch before had been a tuna wrap sandwich made with mayo and oil-packed tuna, which had several hundred calories and double-digit grams of fat. He switched to two sandwiches of ham and cheese with my recommended GG Scandinavian Bran Crispbread, light ham and low-fat cheese (two slices of ham and one piece of cheese per sandwich). This substantial, great-tasting, low-fat lunch gave him 12 grams of fibre and only 235 calories, so he also had a low-cal soup for just 70 calories more. On other days, he'd enjoy a delicious pastrami on rye made with light rye bread (2 slices = 80 calories) and thinly sliced light pastrami (60 calories) and a pickle, topped with mustard, for a total of 150 calories.

At 4 o'clock, instead of cookies from the vending machine (240 calories, double-digit fat grams), he either had an apple (65 calories) with a light-cheese wedge (25 calories), or a dessert made with a cup of Total Yogurt, a few sliced strawberries and a teaspoon of crunchy cereal for just more than 100 calories and no fat.

For his dinner salad, Robb decided he could forgo his usual creamy dressing of almost 300 calories for a teaspoon of olive oil and

Calorienomic Winners: The Favourites of My FoodSmart Clients

So what foods pass the thermogenic test and give you large volume so you never go hungry? What foods when made right have rich taste and texture, and people enjoy them because they're quick and easy to find and prepare? Here are the foodSmart winners most popular with my clients:

- **White-meat fish and seafood:** prawns, crab meat, lobster, scallops, cod, mussels, sole, flounder, skate, snapper
- **Egg whites:** egg white omelettes, plain or with low-calorie cheese or foodSmart vegetables. Less desirable but still acceptable are egg substitutes or adding not more than one yolk.
- **High-calcium dairy foods:** low-fat/fat-free yogurt and milk, low-fat cheese (cottage, ricotta, cream), protein shakes
- **Non-starchy green and white vegetables:** broccoli, green beans, asparagus, artichokes, spinach, lettuce, cauliflower, courgette and cabbage. Vegetables such as these made without oil or butter are free under my programme. And if you like 'fried' vegetables, do them in a nonstick pan with a little chicken stock and olive oil spray or in a George Foreman grill. Vegetable burgers are also good if they're low in carbs.
- **Soups:** made from green and white vegetables and fat-free stock. They fill you up instantly.
- **High-fibre bran crackers** for safe, pre-measured grain, for a fraction of the calories.

This is just a basic list of calorienomic winners. But wait until you see what we do with them in the food chapter, where you'll find as many gourmet main courses as you'll find in any gourmet restaurant in the world.

flavoured balsamic vinegar for just about 40 calories. He had never liked bland steamed vegetables, but now instead of butter, he flavoured them with garlic and herbs and a little spray oil, saving hundreds of calories. And instead of his former main courses of pasta and cheese, or steak or fried chicken – which average 700 to 1,000 calories – he now had prawns with mushrooms and spinach, or grilled filet of sole in a mustard sauce, or my aubergine parmigiana (most of these meals average fewer than 300 calories). And on a night when he wanted dessert, instead of a fruit pie, he had my strawberry shortcake recipe (a wholegrain waffle topped with strawberries and a squirt of light aerosol cream), saving a few hundred calories more and multiple grams of fat.

At 9 p.m., he broke his habit of nibbling all night before bed by having a low-cal chocolate mousse. And on those nights when he stayed up late and wanted a midnight snack, he enjoyed two scoops of my gourmet egg salad on two GG crispbreads for a little more than 100 calories.

There were some weeks when Robb grew so busy at work that he couldn't do his regular gym workout, but he continued to lose weight with variations of this menu.

After 90 days, he walked into my office looking great and smiling: he had lost more than 14 kg (around 30 lb)! 'It's terrific,' he told me. 'I'm never hungry anymore. I have tremendous energy. I have more than enough to eat, and the food is so good. And I'll be able to enjoy my wedding cake totally guilt-free!'

Robb's triumph can be anyone's. Calorienomics is not rocket science. It's a commonsense approach to weight loss that is uncommonly successful for both women and men. It's a triumph of being a selective gourmet and of knowing that weight loss does not mean giving up the pleasure of food.

Calorienomics helps us 'do the numbers' for the life we want and the food control we need. As it trims our calorie budget, it also trims our figures and makes our dining richer.

Those who cannot remember the past
are condemned to wear it.

The Tenth Thin Commandment:
Losing Weight Is Half the Job;
Keeping It Off Is the Other Half

COMMANDMENT ESSENTIALS

- Remember to think historically, not just calorically.
- Keep in mind that even though you've lost the weight, you haven't lost your vulnerability.
- Stick to strategies and planning so you stay in control.
- Throw out all your larger-size clothing.
- Keep problem foods you have a history of abusing out of your house.
- Set a weight ceiling and defend it.
- Keep a photo of yourself at your heaviest weight.
- Keep a food diary.

HAVE YOU EVER HAD A REALLY bad toothache?

One thing it does is give you focus. All you can think of is relieving the pain. You'll even take the day off work or change your entire schedule just to squeeze in a visit to your dentist. You'll endure a large needle's worth of painkiller and hours in the dentist's chair – anything to stop the constant discomfort.

Starting a diet is like that. At first, you're super-motivated. Your weight has made you so uncomfortable that you'll stick with any diet. Mysterious powders, strange foods and an odd eating schedule – you'll do anything to lose the source of your grief.

Warning: as the pounds fade, so does the pain and discomfort that gave you the focus to lose them! If you don't find a way to maintain your new habits, you might find yourself starting all over again.

This is the paradox of weight loss: it may be the only area of human behaviour where success doesn't seem to breed success. Whether it's a business executive closing a big deal or a runner winning a race, their victories inspire them to want more. What is the reason that so many of the winners at losing weight fail to stay in the winner's circle?

They all want to keep the weight off. Hunger and deprivation are clearly not at issue – most maintenance diets offer more calories and much greater variety. It's not a knowledge problem – dieters don't suddenly forget what foods they were eating to keep their calories and carbohydrates low and lose weight. They don't lose sight of the foods they were eating. If that were the case, they could easily refresh their memories by returning to the diet plan or diet book they were following.

Still, there must be a reason why so many people who succeed at losing weight fail at the critical juncture of keeping the weight off. How do we best explain this phenomenon?

What is the winning path through this critical juncture: *weight gain or weight maintain?*

WHY DO SO MANY PEOPLE FLUNK MAINTENANCE?

When you're losing weight, encouragement is ubiquitous. You have an automatic barometer – the scales – to chart your progress and friends and family members to shower you with compliments or an occasional pat on the back. It's easy to stay structured and focused.

But then you hit your desired weight and the well runs dry. The compliments come less frequently. The scales stay in a holding pattern. *On maintenance, it's no longer about the scales dropping but about the scales not going up.* Now, the very real, but less tangible concept of living your life in control of food is the goal.

When someone is losing weight, their body is getting lighter, their clothes are loosening up, and their appearance is improving. The goal is within reach. You think this would be something worth protecting. But as I have shared with you in the pages of this book, human behaviour is often not about logic, but rather *psycho*logic – the logic of the psyche. Sometimes, we don't follow even the most carefully crafted script.

We're all vulnerable to the normal human tendency to let down our guard when we no longer feel threatened. The human psyche is programmed to forget pain. Our minds distance us from unpleasant experiences with the passage of time. It's part of our psychological survival mechanism. So how do you survive on maintenance when the pain and discomfort that inspired weight loss is a thing of the past?

When it comes to weight control, we move away from the very pain and discomfort that motivated us to start dieting. Under these conditions, it's easy to be lulled into thinking that once you lose the weight, your problems are solved. *In truth, it's only by employing successful strategy and winning at maintenance that you can ever really solve the problem.*

The classic diet model suggests that there is a beginning and an end – one that ends with weight loss. *In truth, there may be a beginning and an end to weight loss, but never to weight control.* All the studies show that the winners at weight control don't just lose weight. They make real, tangible changes in their thinking. And the *greatest* change occurs in their approach to maintenance. This is why the word 'diet' comes from the Greek word *dietos*, which means 'way of living'. This is the true meaning of diet and dieting.

Some who flunk maintenance lose the structure of their eating. And what is a diet but a *structured* way of eating? As many people reach their target weight, the gloves come off, and all foods become green lights with only a single admonition: all foods in moderation.

This would be great if we were inclined toward temperance. However, people are not given to moderation but to excess. I would argue that the statement 'all foods in moderation' is more of an idealistic than realistic statement about human behaviour.

In fact, the philosophy of 'all foods in moderation' sets people up to overconsume and flies in the face of research that suggests that too much variety actually encourages overeating. As Tara Parker Pope observed in a recent edition of the *Wall Street Journal*, 'Variety excites the appetite…and stimulates consumption.' Some studies have shown that people who choose from a variety of foods will eat 50 per cent more than those given a single food.

Also, when something tastes great, the tendency is not to moderate but to finish. This is the pleasure principle of the human psyche.

I'm not refuting the 'all foods in moderation' mindset just to be argumentative. I simply want to explain why you may have failed before on maintenance.

A few years ago, the *New York Times* reviewed my work and found that almost 50 per cent of the clients they surveyed had kept off 9–45 kg (20–100 lb) for at least 5 years on maintenance – and I didn't preselect the clients they interviewed. They stated that this success rate stood in marked contrast to the success rate in the field for a 5-year period, which they reported that many experts estimate at around 10 per cent.

When one considers two additional factors, this finding becomes all the more remarkable. Many of these people had not seen me in several years, yet they were still successful. They didn't need to come back for additional visits because they were employing the strategies on their own – techniques you have learned about in this book. The strategies had become for them, as for many of my clients, automatic and easy. Through them, they had found lasting success.

Secondly, the people who come to me from throughout the region of New York, the country and the world have a terrible track record with dieting. Typically, they have tried everything and failed everything. I'm a 'court of last resort' for the 'terminally dieting'. Most of my clients have been to the top weight-control specialists and programmes at universities, teaching hospitals and spas. A very large number of them are privileged to live a life where they select only the best of the best for health care without regard to cost. And yet they have not found success through years and decades of trying with weight programmes – and the best trainers for exercise. Yet, using the strategies of *The Thin Commandments*, years of failure have ended with victory over their weight problems. I am honoured and humbled to have been a part of this victory, for truly they deserve it.

I know of no other programme where so many people have kept off so much weight for so long. If you follow the strategies in this book, you too will reach the winners' circle on maintenance.

Once the weight goes, the Thin Commandments still apply. And for maintenance, in particular, never forget the second one: *think historically, not just calorically.* Forgetting this commandment is perhaps the *greatest* reason why so many who get an 'A' on weight loss flunk maintenance. Many maintainers shift back into caloric thinking alone. The weight is gone and they wonder, 'What's wrong with just a taste of this or that food?'

Well, there's nothing wrong – if they have a history of only being a taster with this or that food. But if they have a history of abusing that food, taking a taste reactivates the craving memory. If you have to fight cravings and hunger every day, how can you expect to control your weight?

WINNING AT MAINTENANCE

The motivation for losing weight is pain and discomfort with your weight. So after the weight evaporates, you need a *shift* in motivation. In fact, a wholesale change in thinking is needed to make the great leap from weight *loss* to weight *control*.

Winners at maintenance let the process be the goal. To live your life in control of food is the process *and* the new goal of maintenance. If you don't have power over food, you'll never be in command of your weight. This is the essence of maintenance!

Successful dieters know they've lost their weight, not their *vulnerability.* Just because you lost 20 or 30 pounds, your taste buds haven't changed. You still have the same number of fat cells. You still have the same personality. *Most important, you still have the same history with the foods that made you heavy!*

Throughout this book, I've used the word *paradox* to clarify a statement that may seem counterintuitive. Perhaps the greatest paradox of all is what I call the paradox of maintenance: *the only way to lose the problem is to realize you never lose the vulnerability.*

Losing weight does not mean that you are any less susceptible to the aroma, taste or texture of certain foods. If you were in the habit of overeating crunchy, salty or sweet-tasting foods before, you'll still be vulnerable to them when you're maintaining your new weight. Whatever started the ball rolling before will start it rolling again. Imagine what can happen if you add 20 different types of foods to your maintenance diet that share these characteristics. You'll be adding a lot of stimulation – and temptation.

Feeling above temptation is a red flag on maintenance. Because the moment you believe you're secure, you run the risk of thinking, 'Why do I need strategies and planning?' That's when the enemy of thin rushes in: complacency. Only by knowing you're being tempted can you resist temptation. *Sometimes the greatest temptation of all is the temptation to become complacent.*

The winners understand that the weight is a symptom of being out of control with certain foods – and certain behaviours. However, it's not the only cause of their problem. The real cause is the food, behaviours – and the thinking. Remember, losing weight is not the equivalent of earning a degree – something you do once and then forget about. Many people believe that losing weight is solving the problem. In truth, it's only half the job.

Keeping it off is the other half.

The Story of Janet

One of my clients, Janet, an executive who had kept weight off for many years, noticed that she was returning to an old habit of stopping for a chocolate bar on the way home from her office. Before long, she was back craving sugar and abusing sweets.

What Janet didn't realize was that eating a chocolate bar on an empty stomach when her blood sugar was low – she often skipped lunch and/or her afternoon snack – was causing her appetite to spiral out of control for the rest of the night.

If Janet had remembered one of the lessons of the Third Command-ment, The Problem May Be in the Food, Not in You, then she would have known that the chemical by-products created when carbohydrates, such as chocolate bars, are burned as fuel stimulate a group of nerve cells in her brain to produce neuropeptide Y, a chemical messenger that made her hungry for even more carbohy-drates and sent her appetite into overdrive.

I pointed out to Janet that eating a chocolate bar at the end of the busi-ness day was the perfect setup for an evening of appetite and sugar cravings. By starting with this chocolate bar

Maintenance: The Importance of Thinking Historically

Like a child let loose in a toy shop, people on maintenance often avail themselves of all the foods the world has to offer. Suddenly, the world is their oyster.

There's just one problem with this approach to maintenance. If they could limit themselves to just a few oysters, they wouldn't have needed a diet to begin with!

To succeed on maintenance, they need fresh guidelines and a new structure based on their own experience with food. This last point is vital. Otherwise, the person might think the new code was being imposed on them from the outside. But when they know the principle is culled from their own history and behaviour – not from some generic eating plan – they feel compelled to honour it.

One of the most critical lessons I've ever learned for success on maintenance is this: *those who honour their history keep it off; those who violate their history fail.*

when her blood sugar was low and her body was craving carbohydrates, she was throwing a match into gasoline. Janet would have been much better off treating herself to a protein meal at a five-star restaurant after a long day because fine food was not her 'issue' – but confectionery was!

If Janet had one of the protein-rich, low-fat yogurts I recommend or a low-fat prawn cocktail, she would have put an abrupt end to her daily blood sugar roller-coaster ride.

This news was a revelation to Janet. She told me, 'Now, I finally realize that it's not about me – that I'm not

lacking motivation or willpower. It's the food I'm choosing that's causing me to spiral out of control again.'

Janet's years of success at weight control did not change her vulnerability to the truth that eating behaviour habituates very quickly or that she is a sugar-sensitive person with a long history of losing control with sweets.

No matter how intelligent you are or how secure you feel, you're no match for the force that is your body's physiological response to a food. *This fact doesn't change just because you're on maintenance.*

Thinking historically, not just calorically, is the new guiding principle.

When a client asks, 'Can I have some peanuts, a chocolate bar or a piece of bread from the breadbasket now that I'm ready for maintenance?' I ask him a simple question in return. 'What is your history with this food or this type of food?' No one has a problem answering this question.

Knowing my clients' histories with food or groups of food gave me insight into their behaviour and the ability to identify potential pitfalls and forks in the road. It was like clearing the field of landmines before the tanks rolled through.

So when one of my clients, a prominent film executive legendary for his negotiating skills with the toughest Hollywood agents, was contemplating a return to breadbaskets, I asked, 'When in your life did you ever negotiate with a breadbasket and win?' Needless to say, he never returned to breadbaskets. And now for the first time, after decades of failure at weight loss, he is succeeding.

By confronting my client with the truth of his own history, he realized that it was easier to live without a destructive habit and that doing so would increase the likelihood of lasting success at weight control. The insight ended his habit of failing at maintenance.

Also, cutting out just one food that was costing him thousands of calories a month gave him freedom to enjoy thousands of other foods – without the fear of gaining weight.

My client's story points out another great truth about maintenance. *True deprivation starts when you return to foods you have a history of abusing because they're certain to rob you of success at weight control.*

10 Tips for Keeping the Weight Off

Here are 9 critical behaviours and 1 additional shift in thinking that make up the 10 most important things to do on maintenance. The first 4 behaviours characterize all my winners. The 6 additional behaviours describe most of my clients. And while I believe that all 10 are important, the first 4 are critical for success.

1. **Wear form-fitting or tight clothes!** When you reach maintenance, you should have one size, and one size only, of

clothing. I've found that *nothing* sounds the warning siren faster or motivates people to act with greater haste than when their clothing gets too tight!

Think about what motivated you to start your diet. If you're like many of my clients, you were uncomfortable with your clothing (or you couldn't fit into it) and appearance. When you have a little extra trouble buttoning a pair of jeans or find it necessary to add an extra notch to your belt, it reawakens the original motivation. When you have only one size, you have no choice but to stay trim. If you save larger sizes, you are making it easy – too easy – to just switch to a larger size instead of acting to correct any errors.

Also, if you don't plan to be heavy again, why save the larger sizes? *When you reach maintenance, throw out the larger sizes – immediately!*

Knowing that you have only one size of clothing adds another powerful incentive to maintain your weight: *economics!* How many of us can afford to buy a whole new wardrobe – especially one in a larger size? Your wallet gives you extra incentive to guard your weight loss.

Before people ever respond to the clarion call to health, they listen to the cry of their clothing getting too tight. I'd have a nearly empty office if I tried to motivate people to stay on maintenance on the basis of health alone.

Your wardrobe is the most powerful deterrent I know of against sliding once more into out-of-control eating. It signals your commitment never to be heavy again. That's why I insist that all maintenance clients discard all clothes that no longer fit, with one exception: I ask them to save the outfit that's their largest size (preferably one they disliked ever having to wear) as an eternal reminder.

2. **Keep problem foods you have a history of abusing out of your home.** *Almost all* the women and a very large percentage of the men I have worked with who regained weight started the slide in their own homes. The slide often began with a food they had a history of abusing but had avoided while they were losing weight.

Remember the study by researchers at the National Weight Control Registry that found that two out of three people who lose weight and keep it off keep problem foods out of their house? Although that food might not tempt you at this moment, I can't urge you strongly enough to remove it from your home or at least keep it permanently out of your sight. Remember, you're always vulnerable to the foods that have tripped you up in the past – even on maintenance. Eventually, people tend to return to their old favourites if they are continually available. On maintenance, even more than weight loss, availability stimulates craving – even if it doesn't happen immediately. Along with keeping only one size of clothes in your house, it's critically important to keep problem foods out of your home.

3. **Set a weight ceiling and defend it.** Pick a number a little above your original goal weight – typically about 1.4 kg (3 lb) for women, 2.2 kg (5 lb) for men – and don't let your weight go above it – ever. No matter what happens, don't let yourself off the hook. Draw a line in the sand. If you see your weight going up, return to the 10-day TurboCharge Diet for several days. When the weight is back down, you can return to maintenance eating. Most of my clients expect increases in weight on weekends because of higher-calorie maintenance meals at home and out. Monday is typically the 'high number' day of the week, but by Friday, they bring the weight back down to their goal weight, by using the foods suggested in my 10-day diet.

4. **Weigh yourself every day.** Your bathroom scales can't weigh your behaviour. However, they will tell you when you gain a pound or two. If you step on the scales the morning after a big meal at a restaurant or special event, your weight could be up. Don't be alarmed. If it's water weight, it will dissipate in 24 to 48 hours. You should expect slight variations during the week.

If it's real weight (1.4 or more kilograms/3 or more pounds that remain over a period of several weeks), that should be a warning to you to take immediate action.

If you find it a bit maddening to follow the daily fluctuations of the scales even though you are eating properly, pick three days of the week on which you will always weigh yourself (for example, Monday, Wednesday and Friday).

5. **Weigh yourself on the Maintenance New Scale,** a nearly foolproof way to predict the scale of tomorrow (see page 184).

6. **Exercise.** It gives you structure and control. It gets you thinking about calorie burn and health consciousness and directs you away from obsessing about food. It's been shown that dieters who exercise regularly succeed the longest at keeping weight off. A study of more than 32,000 dieters by *Consumer Reports* magazine found that 'regular exercise was the number one successful weight-loss maintenance strategy' of more than 81 per cent of the long-term maintainers. In second place, at 74 per cent, was the related strategy of increasing activity in daily routines. Also, as your body becomes lighter, it burns fewer calories. Exercise helps expand your calorie budget by burning the higher-caloric foods of maintenance.

   And remember: exercise generates endorphins, increases energy and elevates mood.

   Exercise provides you with a healthy outlet for stress. These effects help you follow through on your commitments, especially to control your weight. And as an outlet for stress, exercise shortcuts mood eating. It's the perfect alternative to keep your moods out of your foods.

7. **Keep a photo of yourself at your heaviest weight.** For added emphasis, place it next to a picture at your lightest weight. Many of my clients put the photo in a place where they feel most vulnerable – the refrigerator door or kitchen worktop, for example. Others elect to carry the photo in their wallet or purse.

   Some of you may find it upsetting to stare constantly at a picture of yourself at your heaviest weight. Instead, carry a picture of what you look like at your lightest weight. You may find it motivates you even more to protect your accomplishments.

   When it comes to weight control, a picture is truly worth a thousand words.

The Maintenance New Scale

In the first chapter, I spoke about the importance of weighing yourself on the New Scale for Dieting to guarantee that you'd lose weight. I've modified the first chapter New Scale to reflect the new guidelines and thinking necessary for maintenance success.

This simple, 10-question quiz reviews some of the basic skills and attitudes that increase your likelihood of success at weight control. Take this quiz once a week after you reach maintenance. If you answer 'yes' to four of the questions, it's an early warning that you're slipping into bad habits. If you answer 'yes' to five or more questions, you're in danger of regaining the weight – even if your scales haven't started to rise yet. If you see that you're slipping into old ways of thinking or violating your history in some way, just admit it. Evaluate what caused you to slip, the situation and where it might have occurred. See what you can learn from your mistakes so they won't happen again. Remember, slips should teach you, not defeat you.

1. Am I eating any foods that I have a consistent history of abusing?
2. Am I getting sloppy about my behavioural strategies and failing to plan?
3. Am I eating too much of the right foods?
4. Am I nibbling again on whatever foods are around?
5. Am I being negligent about weighing myself regularly and guarding my weight ceiling?
6. Am I keeping problem foods in my house?
7. Am I skipping meals or snacks or going longer than 4 hours without eating?
8. Are my clothes tight?
9. Am I allowing my moods to dictate my foods?
10. Am I skipping exercising frequently during the week?

8. **Keep a food diary.** I'd like you to keep a diary for at least the first 90 days once you are 'on maintenance'. I ask my own clients to keep a diary for a full year. I want them to be certain they can manage the entire cycle of the year, with its holidays, special events, birthdays, summer versus winter eating, and so on. Since the same events and seasons come up year

after year, once you get through the first year, you should be well prepared for the coming ones. After the first year, I frequently ask some clients to continue to keep a food diary or to keep a record of any 'error' such as eating problem foods or excessive quantities of caloric foods.

A diary will serve as a daily reminder of the extras and/or negative eating habits. Writing out your meals and snacks a day in advance will help structure your thinking and help you steer clear of potential trip-ups.

9. **Give yourself clear boundaries.** Boundaries are a strong structure for your eating behaviour. A major study of the winners found that 88 per cent limited some type or classes of food. Another 45 per cent limited the quantities of the foods they ate. Remember, if you don't have a good history of limiting a particular food, avoid it.

I help my clients establish clear boundaries and control their calorie budget by suggesting they stick to lighter menus from Monday through Friday, saving any higher-calorie foods for weekends and special events. This clear boundary helps build an infrastructure of positive behaviours and smart eating habits that becomes automatic after a few weeks.

Most of my winners reinforce their boundaries by continuing to use the techniques of Box It In and Box It Out. Many decide to Box Out a certain category or type of food. For some, it's baked goods, especially breadbaskets. Others avoid sweet baked goods (but may indulge in another type of sweet, such as a chocolate mousse). I want to emphasize again: they don't do this to make their lives difficult or to deprive themselves of something they want. They do it to make it *easier* to succeed at weight control – which is something they want more.

10. **Go beyond the food reward system.** My winners enjoy the pleasure of fine food. Many of them dine regularly at fine restaurants. However, they've evolved beyond the childhood programming that views food as a reward or a treat.

They understand that no matter how beautiful any food looks or how enticing its aroma, if it's a food they have a history of abusing, it's no reward at all.

Some of my clients reward themselves with new clothes. Others enjoy a trip to a spa, a new necklace or a weekend getaway with friends.

These are material rewards. *A far more meaningful reward occurs each morning when they look in the mirror and see a trim body.* There's no greater reward you can give yourself than to live the vision you have for your own life.

RECORDING YOUR OWN INTERNAL VOICE

When I sat down to write this book, I had a goal in mind to share with you every technique I have used to promote success at weight control. Since many studies have shown that staying focused is a key element to weight loss, I make a tape for each of my maintenance clients.

The tapes were designed to reinforce the goals of maintenance and to facilitate the new strategies into their day-to-day living – and to make certain they don't forget the mistakes and lessons of the past. As I've said before, the only way to get permanent weight loss is through permanent changes in your behaviour and eating habits.

My clients find that one of the best ways to guard these changes is to listen to their maintenance tapes. Some listen to their tapes every few weeks. Others listen every day or whenever they need a friendly reminder.

The sample script I've provided you with (see page 188) is similar to the one that's kept my clients focused and successful.

On your tape, you may want to address problems or challenging situations that might be coming up in your life. However, always end your tape on a positive note by speaking to your strengths. Remind yourself that you have the intelligence, not the food. Also, make a note to yourself that if you're upset or disappointed, that 'it's not about the food'. Every time you eat in response to life's disappointments, you give up power over your own destiny. Happy, sad, rich or poor – it's still better being thin. Or should I say 'staying thin'.

The 10 Biggest Maintenance Busters

Successful weight control extends beyond knowing what strategies work best. It's also about learning to appreciate the forces that can chip away at your resolve and long-term success.

I've identified the top 10 maintenance busters. They may not lead to failure immediately, but over time, they erode your control and healthy new eating habits.

1. **Skipping meals.** Special bulletin: a new study indicates that the number one behaviour that leads people to gain weight is skipping meals!

   Perhaps the greatest maintenance mistake is skipping meals or going too long without eating. This habit, which some people engage in to lose weight, will cause your blood sugar to dip and can increase your appetite and cravings.

   Some people are trained to believe that if they eat three meals a day, they'll be fine. You can eat three meals and still go too long without eating because there are too many hours in between meals and snacks. Some people decide to skip lunch or, worse, breakfast. Others neglect to have the required late-afternoon snack. On maintenance, missing this snack is the equivalent of skipping a meal.

   If you have lunch at noon and don't eat dinner until 7, you've gone too long without eating (remember Janet's story on page 178). This will make it more likely that you'll overeat at dinner or fall prey to night-eating syndrome.

2. **Nibbling.** There are few things that can undo your control and the structure of your eating habits faster than mindlessly picking or nibbling on foods you have a history of abusing or picking on whatever foods you happen to encounter in the course of a day.

   Worse, most people don't count what they nibble and pick on toward their calorie budget. Nibbling is like a cancer that insidiously eats away at your calorie budget.

   Once you grant yourself permission to eat whatever's in your environment, everything becomes fair game. Slowly, the calories start going up while your control starts heading south.

Sample Tape: Maintenance

These are some of the major themes I use on my clients' tapes, which I've found to be the most powerful and help produce the greatest success on maintenance. Not all these statements may apply to you, so pick the ones that resonate the most, or create new ones just for your lifestyle – and your history!

- Losing weight is half the job; keeping it off, the other half.
- 'My new goal is one day at a time, to live my life in control with food and to avoid any foods and behaviours that weaken my control (list any negative foods or behaviours). There is no food I can't have. There are foods I may choose not to have because they don't work for me.'

- 'I have lost my weight but not my vulnerability, so I need to stay focused.'
- 'I didn't come this far to take orders from a piece of food.'
- Think historically, not just calorically.
- Remind yourself that this way of living is an infant in your life and needs nurturing.
- Remind yourself of the trigger foods and behaviours that each time you returned to, you gained back your weight. If you have trigger foods you have Boxed Out, remind yourself of them and the mantra 'I don't take the first little taste; I don't begin; I don't have any problems.' Reiterate for your psyche: 'The first taste is not about the calories but the cravings. I

Nibbling becomes a habit that can quickly become as addictive as any drug.

The three meals and two or three snacks on my eating plan give you structure. Nibbling destroys that structure. Remember, finger control is the essence of weight control – unless you're nibbling one of the 'free foods' such as green and white vegetables (which I will explain in the diet chapter). Once you go back to nibbling on whatever food(s) happen to be lying around, you sacrifice eating structure.

On maintenance, it's critical to keep clear boundaries with nibble foods. Don't deviate unless it's a planned indulgence with a fixed amount of food. And avoid eating with your fingers unless you choose a low-calorie food from my eating don't reactivate cravings.'

- Remind yourself of challenging situations that might be coming up or any problems you may be having with food or your eating behaviour.
- 'This work is not about dieting but about the quality of my life.'
- 'This work is not about deprivation, but liberation: liberation from a lifetime of weight problems and failing again and again with my weight on maintenance.'
- 'If I choose to avoid a certain food, it's not that I can't have it. I avoid it because it doesn't work for me.'
- 'If I'm not planning, I'm planning to fail.'
- 'I need to stay focused, otherwise, I'll be focused on why I'm heavy and miserable. One way or the other, this will be on my mind each day, but now I'm on the winning side, and I plan to stay there.'
- 'I deserve to be trim. I deserve to succeed at this. I deserve to be in control of my life with food.'
- Complacency is the enemy of thin – stay focused.
- 'I think like a winner – to be trim and successful is my greatest treat, goodie and dessert.'
- 'I have intelligence; a piece of food doesn't.'
- 'I'm finally free to live the vision I have for my own body.'
- 'Finally, I have a new taste: the taste of thin, the taste of success. This is worth protecting!'

plan, such as the fruit, crudités, or my own recommended bran crackers.

3. **Eating too much of the right foods.** After weeks or months on a diet, people are generally more aware of the types of foods they're eating. However, they're often not as aware of the *quantity* of the foods they're eating.

   Many of my clients have got into trouble eating too much of the 'right foods' such as chicken, beef, and even fruit – particularly when they're nibbling from bowls of cut-up fruit or bowls of grapes and cherries. Some ate too much because it was 'healthy' food, and they assumed that portion size didn't matter. Others got into hot water when they ate what they thought was only a single serving, when it was actually two or three times that amount. (This typically happens in restaurants, especially with pasta dishes.) To correct for this, just have pasta as an appetizer.

There's a tendency on maintenance to let quantity fly under the radar. But it can contribute thousands of extra calories to your diet. When a client tells me she's following the protocol, but still gaining weight, I often suspect that the culprit is too much of the right foods.

4. **Reactivating cravings.** There's a popular misconception in the field of weight control that the way to eliminate a craving is to eat the food you're longing. For some who don't have a history of compulsive eating or have never abused that food, this may be true. For the rest of us, eating foods we have a long history of abusing (such as trigger foods) does not satisfy cravings — it fuels them.

If you think that just tasting a food you've decided to Box Out is not *calorically significant*, you're right. However, from a control point of view, you're dead wrong. Any time you stir up interest or reactivate cravings in a food you've elected to avoid, you give your psyche a green light. Once you tell yourself it's okay to have a little, you're inviting temptation and overconsumption. You start looking for the food again, you start thinking about it and you start noticing it more, or worse, you start buying it and keeping it around your home — even though it's a food you have a non-history of being a 'taster' with and a long history of excessively abusing.

5. **Letting the supplies of healthy food run out.** Even my most well-intentioned maintenance clients have run into problems because they overlooked a simple but key ingredient for success. You can't construct a building without the right tools. Similarly, you'll never succeed at maintenance if you don't have enough of the right foods.

After some of my clients get to the goal, they stop buying the foods that contributed to their success. They become careless about stocking their homes with the right foods. It's not that they don't like these foods or intended to stop eating them. Since the goal has been achieved, buying the right, or should I say 'calorienomic winners', no longer seems paramount. They soon start eating the higher-caloric foods that are around the house for others. Another danger is that they stop stocking their ThinPack and carrying it with them, and they end up eating whatever foods happen to be around in meeting rooms or when they travel. Before too long, this becomes the new habit.

6. **The add-on effect.** On maintenance, I often see people continually adding new foods to their diet without attempting to balance their calorienomic books. Even if you choose healthy foods such as wholemeal bread, brown rice and fruit, you need to balance your budget by subtracting or substituting for the extra foods you add.

Simply because you're excluding or limiting foods you have a history of abusing doesn't mean you can add one new food after another to your diet. When a maintenance client asks if she can add a new food, and I see that her weight is stable, I remind her that her body doesn't need any extra calories. So, if she wants to add a new food(s) today, I ask her what she's willing to subtract from her calorie budget tomorrow. Or, I'll tell her to add a couple of extra days of light eating to her diet. On maintenance, people tend to practise 'one-way mathematics' – only addition. They forget about subtraction, substitution or division. Watch for this maintenance buster; it often eludes notice.

7. **Returning to mood eating.** You can lose all the weight you want, but if you run to food the next time you're upset, you're jeopardizing your chances for lasting success on maintenance.

Sometimes when people are losing weight, they refuse to eat – even if something bothers them (demonstrating that they clearly have the power to control mood eating), since they are determined to lose weight each week. Once they've lost the weight, it's easy for them to slip back into the old habit of eating every time they're anxious or annoyed. Yet, they will be a lot more upset if they start losing control and regaining the weight.

Feeling in control in your own life can be a bulletproof vest against the slings and arrows of life's annoyances and misfortunes. Sometimes success on maintenance is not about your foods, but your moods. Stay alert!

8. **Creep syndrome.** People don't go to bed trim and wake up heavy. Weight gain is a slow, subtle process that often goes undetected. Most people don't get too alarmed if they gain back a pound or two. Or, they rationalize. You might hear, 'It's only a few pounds, so it's not a big deal.' Before too long, those 2 pounds have morphed into 3, and that same person says, 'It's just 3 pounds.' And the 3 becomes 5, 8 and then 10.

   This is why I insist that you set a weight ceiling, guard it, and make no excuses. And if that number starts to go up, take action! Before you even realize it, those 5 or 6 pounds can turn into 15 or even 20.

9. **Failing to plan.** Planning is about protectiveness. When you start a diet, the desire to lose the weight and look and feel better pushes you to plan. After you lose the weight, you may believe there's nothing left to protect and, therefore, no urgent need to plan.

   You may stop carrying your ThinPack, or find yourself going to restaurants hungry, or going food shopping when you're most vulnerable.

   Often, failing to plan goes undetected. It can take the form of something as benign as sitting near an open bowl of nuts or not moving the breadbasket out of arm's reach. Even these subtle planning blunders can have a *dramatic* effect on your cravings over time – and your success at maintenance.

   Losing weight does not reduce the need for planning. Actually, planning makes things easier because it guards your success. It helps you avoid pitfalls and establish boundaries.

   Remember, if you fail to plan, you're planning to fail.

10. **Tomorrowisms.** 'I'll do it tomorrow. Just not now.' Does this sound familiar? It's the promise of someone who sees that they're gaining weight back but puts off going back on their diet.

It's also a reflection of what I like to call *maintenance resistance*. Once someone grows accustomed to the greater variety on maintenance, they often resist returning to lighter food even if their weight starts going up.

If you know that you're prone to maintenance resistance, it's important to act quickly. When it's just a few pounds, you can take off these pounds typically in a week or 10 days. So even if you're resistant, you don't have to push yourself for too long. The longer you delay, the more your weight goes up, the longer it will take to get it off, and the more maintenance resistance increases. Also, your weight is increasing because you're eating too many calories and returning to negative eating habits. If you're returning to old habits, it's important to end them quickly, not to keep reinforcing them through delay.

To help you do this, write out a day or week's eating plan in advance. Tell yourself, 'If I stick to this, I'll lose X amount of weight.' Also, try ridding your home of any foods that might be tempting you to eat incorrectly.

If you're still having trouble or find you can't do it alone, enlist a friend who also wants to lose weight, and give each other mutual support, join a weight programme or contact an online support group, such as ediet.com. Many of my clients also find that going to a spa or health farm for a few days or a week gets them away from trigger foods and unhealthy eating habits and jump-starts their motivation. I often send my clients to quality spas to recharge.

Don't be a passive observer when you see negative behaviour.

Remember, the more you say 'tomorrow', the more you'll weigh tomorrow.

These 10 maintenance busters don't require much interpretation. However, the insouciant, devil-may-care attitude of some is more subtle and creates a fertile breeding ground for problems. When you realize that *the process is the goal* – to live your life in control of food – that your maintenance journey is just beginning, I believe you'll appreciate the need to protect and not to 'test yourself' or the boundaries.

When a client says to me, 'I just wanted to test myself', I smile and remind him that the reason he's sitting in my office is that he already tried to test himself – and flunked. And if that attitude persists, he'll be a perfect candidate for flunking maintenance.

THE ONLY COMPLIMENT YOU'LL EVER NEED TO HEAR

There is only one way to achieve permanent weight loss, and that is to make a lasting change in your eating habits. This is the truth. It would be far easier for me to say to each of you, 'All foods in moderation.' And that's what I would wish for all people. But as I've said throughout this chapter, that's not the behaviour of all people. The statement 'all foods in moderation' is only for those who are given to moderation and whose history bears this out. For the rest of us, strategy comes first.

If you follow the strategies in this commandment, one thing is certain: you'll do maintenance in a new way and get a fresh result – success. Most important, you'll hear the compliment most dieters never hear – 'You've kept it off!'

Then you'll know you've not only lost the weight, *you've also lost the problem.*

PART II

THE THIN
COMMANDMENTS
DIET

The Eating Plan

WHY CHOOSE THIS DIET?

Throughout my career, I've experimented with countless diets. The one I am about to share with you represents the core of the diet I put my clients on. Most of the people who come to me for advice want to lose weight quickly and safely. The 10-day TurboCharge Diet fulfils these criteria – and more. It produces quick weight loss and is easy to follow, but it also gives the most volume, and prevents hunger and cravings, all while offering great-tasting, low-calorie foods.

Time and time again, so many of my clients, particularly women, complained they couldn't lose more than a few pounds on other diets. How is it that this diet has worked for them?

I believe it's my diet's synergistic combination of foods that literally turbocharges your body's capacity to lose weight that makes all the difference. The selection of foods it includes come from my own observations and from countless hours spent sifting through thousands of pages of scientific studies, many of which, I believe, will influence diets in decades to come.

In the Ninth Commandment, Treat Your Calories Like Money, I spoke of the power of certain foods to promote greater weight loss over foods of equal calories. This part of the book will further explore the weight-loss benefits of three special foods – and one food group with a magic mineral – that will help you jump-start your weight loss and keep it off for a lifetime. First, you'll learn why I call seafood the 'Concorde to Thin' and why it's one of the best choices for *rapid* weight loss, satiety, superior nutrition, and looking younger and living longer. You'll also find out about the weight-control benefits of the spice cinnamon and how it regulates the hunger hormone insulin and may help you in losing weight – and even lowering your bad cholesterol. Yet it has no calories, and it tastes great. I've also found cinnamon helpful in keeping sugar cravings at bay.

Next, I'll explain why high-fibre foods are so effective at diminishing appetite and why GG Scandinavian Bran Crispbread may be the crown jewel of this group. It's such a great appetite suppressant that I call it the 'hunger killer'. You'll also discover that by simply eating foods rich in the mineral calcium, specifically dairy foods, you might be able to increase your weight loss by 70 per cent.

Through this synergistic combination of foods, along with the recommended amount of water and suggested menus, you'll be able to eat more while taking in fewer calories – as well as lose more weight. *Who said a calorie is just a calorie?*

This section also gives you sound, practical guidelines for handling planned splurges, a way to reduce facial bloat in just 10 days, and advice on what to do if you've reached a weight-loss plateau. Crucially, it also offers suggestions and guidelines to keep that weight off permanently. Most of all, the advice in this section will make it easy for you to join the ranks of the winners at weight control. So, what are you waiting for?

FOUR FOODS THAT GIVE YOU AN UPPER HAND AT WEIGHT LOSS

Have you ever heard someone talk about a great poker player? Typically, they'll say something to the effect of 'That guy just can't lose. He's probably got an ace up his sleeve.' In other words, he's got an edge – an advantage that virtually guarantees him the winning hand.

I believe that those of you embarking on this diet also have an edge. But instead of having just one ace up your sleeve like a star poker player, you have four. That's right. You have four aces that just might help you reach your target weight and keep that weight off for a lifetime.

As I mentioned in the introduction to this section, the diet emphasizes three foods and one food group with a magic mineral, all of which allow you to keep the taste without the calories. Now, I'll explain to you what they are and why they just might put you, as they've put thousands of my clients, on the short path to rapid, safe weight loss.

Why Seafood Is the 'Concorde to Thin'

Think about the last meal you ate. Did it leave you satisfied, or did you find yourself thinking about eating or reaching for more food a short time later? Many things influence how much you eat, and now research is showing that satiety may be one of the most important factors. Simply, satiety is the feeling of fullness or satisfaction that occurs when your stomach and intestine signals your brain that you've had enough. If you want to shed weight quickly while reducing your waistline, it's not just the amount but also the type of food you choose that may matter the most.

For as long as I can remember, I've championed seafood, especially prawns and fish, and called it the 'Concorde to Thin' a decade ago in my book *Thin Tastes Better*. Now, it appears that scientific evidence may prove me right. Seafood has always been one of the very best sources of low-calorie, vitamin-rich, nutrient-dense protein and may also be one of the best choices if you're looking to fill up faster, control hunger, and *ultimately* lose weight at an optimal rate – even if you've been unable to lose weight on other diets.

Fish gets the highest marks on the 'Satiety Index', a way of measuring how full people feel during a 2-hour period after eating 240 calories worth of food, developed by obesity expert Susanne Holt, PhD. The more protein, fibre, or water a food has, the more it satisfies.

On Dr Holt's index, *fish came in second overall to boiled potatoes as the most satisfying food per calorie and was the only protein source at the top of the list.* Since most varieties of finfish and shellfish provide between 100 to 200 calories per 100 g (3½ oz), based on the Satiety Index, they're among the best choices if you're looking to fill up and feel satisfied. Bulky high-fibre foods, such as fruits, grains and vegetables, also rate high. But they can't compare to fish. Needless to say, many baked goods, including biscuits and cakes, finish near the bottom, because 240 calories worth is often a small portion of these foods.

Based on the 240-calorie ceiling, you could have 200 g (7 oz) of prawns, 21 medium-size scallops, 150 g (5½ oz) of salmon, or 1.1 kg (2½ lb) of mussels (in the shell). Assuming, of course, you could eat that much at one sitting!

Dr Holt's findings support what I've taught for years – that a key to controlling weight is to eat foods that have fewer calories per gram, so you ultimately leave the table satisfied without blowing your calorie budget.

Dr Virend K. Somers, PhD, a professor of medicine in the division of cardiovascular disease and hypertension at the Mayo Clinic, and a man whose scientific work I admire greatly, has a theory about why fish may be one of the best foods for weight loss.

Dr Somers says that fish may influence your body's production of *leptin*, a hormone manufactured by your fat cells and secreted by your fat tissue. In people, leptin is a satiety factor and acts on the hypothalamus, the part of your brain that regulates appetite. The level of leptin circulating in your bloodstream, says Dr Somers, is often directly proportional to the amount of body fat, or adipose tissue, you have. For example, women generally have more body fat than men and tend to manufacture more leptin. Researchers at Rockefeller University found that the amount of leptin correlates to how much fat is stored in the body. Higher leptin levels are found in people with more fat and reduced levels in those who dieted.

Dr Somers believes that fish 'may change the relationship between leptin and body fat, *making the body more sensitive to leptin's message of satiety*'. Perhaps this is why fish is the only protein at the top of the Satiety Index.

This heightened sensitivity to leptin's satiety message may have critical applications to helping you lose weight without ever feeling hungry. Earlier in this book, I discussed how the protein *neuropeptide Y* – described in one study as 'the most powerful appetite stimulant yet discovered' – increases food intake – especially for carbohydrates – and stimulates secretion of insulin and cortisol, which can lead to fat accumulation. Leptin may counteract the effects of neuropeptide Y. Leptin may also offset the effects of anandamide, another powerful feeding stimulant, and promote

The Benefits of Fish

Fish offers so many positives for dieters that it's hard to list them all in one sitting. However, the following are a few you might want to know about:

- Fish is nutrient dense, meaning it offers large amounts of protein and significant minerals and vitamins without a lot of calories and saturated fat.
- The protein in fish is easily digested.
- Fish contains small amounts of fat (most types contain less than 5 per cent). Even higher fat varieties, such as salmon, still have less than 15 per cent, which is lower than most cuts of meat. Fish is also lower in saturated fat than many other protein sources, such as chicken and turkey.
- Fresh fish, not canned, is generally low in sodium. Most varieties of fish contain 60 to 100 milligrams

per 100 g (3½ oz). Excess salt can contribute to bloat and increase your blood pressure.

- Fish leaves you feeling more satisfied after a meal.
- Fish is loaded with unsaturated fatty acids, called omega-3 fatty acids. Omega-3 fatty acids are one of two types of essential fatty acid – the other being omega-6 fatty acids – that our bodies can't manufacture on their own and can only be derived from food. Some studies have shown that omega-3 fatty acids may improve our cells' sensitivity to insulin, thereby reducing our chances of developing excess body fat. These same fatty acids may also increase thermogenesis, so that more of the calories from your food are burned up during digestion instead of being stored.

the synthesis of α-MSH, an appetite suppressant. The result: lower food intake. A Purdue University study found that leptin may inhibit the synthesis of fat in fat cells and increase the burning of fat in muscle cells.

Leading nutritional researcher Michael Zemel, PhD, has observed that leptin 'decreases appetite and increases metabolism'. *When it comes to having a meal, fish may be the ultimate calorienomic food for decreasing appetite, giving large volume and low calories, and turbocharging your body's capacity to lose weight. In fact, fish may stand alone in the entire world of food in offering these benefits for your success at weight loss.*

Cinnamon – A Simple Way to Spice Up Weight Loss

In your wildest dreams, could you conjure up a delicious, zero-calorie food that may help you control your hunger, lose weight and possibly even encourage the development of your lean muscle mass? If you thought, even for a moment, that such a food existed, would you frantically search the Internet or scour the globe to find it? Fortunately, you may not have to resort to such measures. More than likely, you'll locate this food during a 5-minute visit to your local supermarket. How's that for quick and easy?

If you've eaten a baked apple or piece of French toast in the past week, you may have enjoyed cinnamon and didn't even realize it. Many of you know that cinnamon tastes great on a variety of foods, but what you may *not* know is that cinnamon may be one of the best foods for weight loss. It turns out that consuming just ½ teaspoon of ground cinnamon daily may help control your hunger, keep your waistline in check, and even help you gain more lean muscle. Does this all sound too good to be true? Well, it isn't, at least according to Richard A. Anderson, PhD, lead scientist at the Beltsville Human Nutrition Research Center in Maryland and an authority on the effects of food on human metabolism.

To start, says Dr Anderson, cinnamon improves insulin activity in fat cells. When you eat a meal, your pancreas releases insulin (a protein), which prompts your cells to take in the glucose (sugar) floating in your bloodstream. Fat cells, notes Dr Anderson, utilize sugar. So the more excess sugar you have, the more fuel your fat cells have. In other words, your fat cells start getting fatter. Cinnamon makes your cells use insulin more efficiently, thereby increasing sugar metabolism – a process by which your cells convert blood sugar to energy. By limiting the amount of sugar in your blood, you're depriving your fat cells of their sole source of food. Dr Anderson's latest research shows that cinnamon cuts blood-sugar levels by 20 to 30 per cent.

To control your weight, you need to keep your blood-sugar levels stable. As Dr Anderson so adroitly noted, 'Whenever there's a problem with someone's weight, there's often a problem with his or her sugar.'

Cinnamon may aid weight management by helping control hunger. Simple sugars, such as the type found in biscuits and white bread, require relatively little time to digest and cause a rapid rise in your blood-glucose levels. When this happens, your pancreas produces a corresponding amount of insulin, so your blood-sugar levels don't go through the roof. This large, rapid insulin response often causes your blood sugar to fall too low just a short time after the biscuit or bread is finished. Before long, you may find you're hungry for something else. Typically, you'll reach for more biscuits or a similar food to get your blood sugar back up. 'Since cinnamon helps control the amount of insulin your body needs, it ultimately controls satiety. If you're not hungry all the time, you'll take in fewer calories,' says Dr Anderson.

In my own work, I have used cinnamon very effectively to help control sugar cravings and found it to be particularly helpful for lessening PMS cravings. Many of my clients have used cinnamon as a creative strategic tool to put a quick end to carbohydrate bingeing with baked goods and bread products. *It is a powerful tool for your error correction and containment in the arsenal of the strategies you have learned in this book.*

Most significant, cinnamon may help you lose weight by increasing your body's production of lean muscle mass. Because cinnamon helps increase sugar metabolism, it frees up insulin to perform one of its other important jobs: lean muscle development. Insulin controls the uptake of amino acids (the building blocks of protein) into muscles, which increases the synthesis of muscle protein. 'When insulin doesn't have to spend a lot of time controlling your blood-sugar levels, it can spend more time converting amino acids into protein, which leads to increased lean body mass,' says Dr Anderson. By adding cinnamon to your diet, it may be possible to lose weight without decreasing lean muscle mass.

A central goal of my eating plan is weight control and fat loss. In which case, a good long-term solution is one that improves insulin sensitivity, controls hunger and promotes the development of lean muscle. Cinnamon just might do all three.

Dr Anderson's findings confirm what I've observed firsthand in my work – that cinnamon augments flavour while simultaneously enhancing satiety. Frequently, foods that improve taste stimulate cravings. Cinnamon seems to do the opposite. I've also found that cinnamon helps turn off sugar cravings and restores blood-sugar levels after too much carbohydrate bingeing.

As an added bonus for your health, cinnamon may lower total

cholesterol, bad cholesterol and triglycerides anywhere from 13 to 30 per cent. That's comparable to the benefits seen with statin drugs. Dr Anderson says that boiling one cinnamon stick in a cup of water to make coffee or tea will give you the same effect as ½ tablespoon of ground cinnamon.

Volumize with Fibre

Eat more fibre. You've probably heard that advice before. But do you know why you should eat more fibre?

Fibre has many functions, but it is probably best known for its ability to relieve and prevent constipation. But what you may not know is that high-fibre foods, especially my GG Scandinavian Bran Crispbread and the green and white vegetables on the diet, offer three big benefits for people looking to lose weight, as leading nutrition writer Jane Brody recently observed in her weekly column in the *New York Times*. 'They hold water in the gut and take longer to digest, and some of their calories are eliminated unabsorbed. In other words, they can fill you up before they fill you out.'

To start, your body absorbs fewer calories from foods high in fibre because your digestive enzymes can't break fibre down, which means that your body can't absorb it. This is why high-fibre foods, provided they are low in fat, also tend to be low in calories.

Since your body absorbs so little fibre, many researchers now say the grams of fibre in a food can be subtracted from the total grams of carbohydrates in the food. This results in a net carb count, meaning you count only those carbohydrates that have a tangible effect on your blood sugar. To be 'carb smart' means to choose foods that have a favourable ratio to fibre (vegetables, for example) and to avoid the ones that don't (such as croissants, processed breads, pasta).

Many high-fibre foods allow you to engage in an activity I have described as *volumizing*. Simply put, *volumizing allows you to eat large amounts of food while taking in fewer calories*. Certain fibre-rich foods provide a lot of volume, or size, for the calories, so you can eat more of them without packing on extra weight from the calories.

Equally important, high-fibre foods make a meal feel larger (partially because they bulk up after they enter your stomach) and remain longer in your stomach, so you stay full longer. Since it can also take up to 24 hours for high-fibre foods to pass through your

Opticarb Eating

As I said earlier in this book, *opticarbs* are foods that promote weight loss by accelerating your body's ability to lose weight while also tending to eliminate the hunger and cravings that sabotage success on so many diets.

The eating plan draws on cutting-edge research to include a select group of foods that work synergistically to optimize the body's ability to lose weight, even in those most resistant to weight loss.

This group of foods is further enhanced by what I call the opticarbs – a unique group of low-carbohydrate foods that promote *success* at weight control by:

1. Enhancing your body's ability to lose weight so that you lose significantly more weight on a diet that includes these carb foods over a diet with other carb foods of equal calories.
2. Controlling hunger and cravings, especially for the 'bad carbs' – high-glycaemic carbohydrate foods that cause fast, dramatic spikes in your blood sugar, which may, in turn, contribute to weight gain.
3. Providing you with generous volume and superior nutrition for relatively few calories.

These 'smart-carb' foods include:

- High-calcium dairy products, especially yogurt, high-calcium dairy shakes, and low-fat/skimmed cheese and milk.

- Green and white, low-starch vegetables, such as cucumber, spinach, broccoli, cabbage, asparagus, mushrooms, celery, salad greens and green peppers, which give volume and fibre for appetite control and satiety, plus super nutrition. These vegetables are so low in calories and carbs that you can include them as free foods.

- GG Scandinavian Bran Crispbread. The GG is the only grain that gives your body 0.0 'net' carbs, while supplying more fibre and fewer calories (and fewer carbs) per ounce than other grains.

- Grapefruit – the only fruit with carbs that has been demonstrated to accelerate the body's capacity to lose weight.

It is this mosaic of foods that I call opticarb eating. These are the carbs that promote success at weight loss. You get the carbs without the consequences!

digestive tract, they can help control your appetite – and calorie intake – for up to a day. Similarly, fibre also slows down nutrient absorption after a meal, thereby controlling your blood sugar and reducing the amount of insulin your body needs. Large volumes of food activate stretch receptors in your stomach, which then send a signal to your brain that you feel full. To activate these receptors faster, you're better off with foods that provide large portions with low calories, since the number of calories you consume has far less impact on satiety than volume. For example, 100 g (3½ oz) of brown rice equals about 115 calories; but a 100-calorie serving of fibre-rich, garlic-roasted broccoli will give you a serving of 375 g (13 oz). Which do you think is going to fill up you up faster?

Finally, many fibre-rich foods, such as broccoli and asparagus, require more time to chew, which gives your body more time to register when you're no longer hungry, so you're less likely to overeat.

Lose Your Carb Face in 10 Days

Shakespeare said: 'God has given you one face, and you make yourself another.'

The face tells all. For most of us, the part of our bodies that shows the first signs of weight gain and bloat or weight loss is the face. While many of my clients complain that they can't fit into their clothes or complain about wanting to lose their belly fat, what really shows up first is weight gain in their faces. If you've ever looked closely at a person who has put on a significant amount of weight or has binged on carbohydrates, his face often looks puffy and distended. This is what some of us who work in the field of weight management call the 'carb face'.

There are a lot of things that can cause you to acquire a carb face. As luck would have it, some of the foods we love the most are the worst thing for our appearance. In particular, refined carbohydrates, especially those found in baked goods, some crackers, breads and pasta, may cause your body to retain fluid. In fact, for every gram of carbohydrates you take in, your body tends to retain 3 to 5 grams of water. Many of these products also contain excess salt, which may compound facial bloat. Most refined carbohydrates are also high on the glycaemic index, a scale that rates foods according to their impact on blood-sugar levels. High-glycaemic foods are digested quickly and flood your bloodstream with glucose. When-

Some of you reading this may be curious why I've made no mention of grains, which are by all known standards an excellent source of fibre. While I do like some grains – specifically the GG Scandinavian Bran Crispbread – and include them in my diet, I've found that they may not be the best choice for dieters. For one, grains do not provide the one thing you want most: volume at low calories (which you can see from the previous example of brown rice compared with broccoli). Indeed, if the goal is to put more food on your plate, why limit yourself to tiny portions of brown rice and whole-wheat pasta, when you can have large portions of foods such as spinach sautéed with garlic and ginger, two steamed artichokes topped with a tablespoon of fat-free salad dressing, or Dr G's Light Pizza on two GGs for fewer calories – and fewer carbohydrates?

Portion control is another problem with grains. I've found that people tend to overeat grain-based foods – even healthy choices like

ever that much sugar is present in your bloodstream, your body responds by releasing insulin to bring your blood-sugar levels back to normal. When sugar increases insulin levels in the body, more calories and fat are stored.

The good news about following this diet is that it not only reduces your weight, but it can also close the door on facial bloat. If you follow the 10-Day TurboCharge Diet, with its abundance of low-carbohydrate foods, many of which are rich in skin-friendly DMAE, you'll see a great improvement in your bloated carb face. Just as the face is the first to show weight gain, the reverse is also true. It's also the first part of your body to show weight loss when you follow the

right type of diet. Remember to drink plenty of water to facilitate the process.

I've often said that your clothing is the first line of defence to keep you from gaining weight. You might want to think of your face as the second battalion. If you've ever had a night of carbohydrate bingeing, you may notice the next day that your face looks puffy. Reducing facial bloat will accentuate the appearance of your weight loss, making it appear as though the weight is literally melting away. My clients tell me that the first thing they notice after going on the 10-Day TurboCharge Diet is a reduction in their facial bloat. It immediately makes them look trimmer.

brown rice and other whole grains, especially when served in restaurants or in unmeasured quantities. I don't mean to disparage grain products. Provided they're not fried or prepared in oil and you don't have a history of abusing them, they can be helpful. But in terms of calories per ounce, you'll do much better with green vegetables. Alternatively, get your fill of grains, as my clients do, from the GG Scandinavian Bran Crispbread, which gives volume, crunch, satiety and low calories.

What to Do if You're Doing Everything Right But Still Not Losing Weight

It doesn't happen very often. But every once in a while, a client will tell me that he's honouring his history, using good strategy, following the diet – and still not losing weight. Sometimes, it's the seemingly innocuous amounts of food you unconsciously put in your mouth during the day that, over time, add the extra weight. For instance:

- A mother might help herself to a few chips or the last few bites of a sandwich, or eat several spoonfuls of pasta her toddler couldn't finish. It may seem hardly worth the effort to refrigerate such a small amount, and why let it go to waste? That is, of course, until you realize that those three or four spoonfuls could add up to an extra 150 calories.
- You've just come to the end of a box of cereal and notice that a few tablespoons have spilled into the bottom

of the box. Why, you might think, let it go to waste or spend the effort returning it to the cupboard? Well, those few tablespoons could add a few hundred calories to your breakfast.

- You go food shopping and help yourself to a small sample of cheese and crackers. No problem, right? Except that cheese and crackers could end up costing you 150 to 200 calories (a 2-cm/1-in cube of regular Cheddar cheese contains about 110 calories).
- You're whipping up a batch of chocolate chip cookies for your son's football team and find there are a 'few' spoonfuls left at the bottom of the mixing bowl. One spoonful equals a single, medium-size cookie, and you just ate four (300 calories).
- You're sitting at a bar, waiting to meet a friend for dinner and decide

Lose Up to 70 Per Cent More Weight with Calcium

There's an expression, 'Don't cry over spilled milk.' Well, if you knew what dairy products could do to turbocharge your weight loss, you just might shed a tear or two the next time a glass of milk hits the floor. And this isn't the latest fad; it's real science. At least according to leading nutrition researcher Michael Zemel, PhD, chairman of the nutrition department at the University of Tennessee.

In a 6-month study, Dr Zemel discovered that people whose

to help yourself to a 'small' handful of peanuts before she arrives. That handful of nuts could be costing you anywhere from 200 to 300 calories.

- You go to Starbucks each day for a jumbo coffee, forgetting that adding extra milk, or worse, cream may have just upped the calorie count of your drink 25 to 30 per cent.
- You're dining at your favourite restaurant, and the waiter brings you a dressed salad with a *few* croutons on top. That tablespoon of garlic croutons has 86 calories and 3.5 grams of fat. The salad dressing may have a few hundred calories.

Does any of this sound familiar? As you can see, these little bites of food can add many calories to your diet and possibly several inches to your waistline. What's even worse, they can easily start a daily pattern of 'little extras'. Fortu-

nately, it's not too difficult to avoid these mystery calories. The following are a few of my favourite strategies to help tilt the scales back in your favour.

- **Keep a journal or diary.** Writing down the foods you eat is a good way to avoid those little nibbles that add extra calories. In your diary, circle any foods made with sauces, oils, or those containing extra quantities. You might cut back on the nibbling because you simply get tired of writing down everything you eat.
- **Carry your ThinPack.** Take a few healthy, low-calorie snacks, such as a few GG crackers or an apple, with you so you won't have to give in to higher-calorie temptations.
- **Never cook or go into food situations hungry.** You're more likely to overeat or give in to a food you have a history of abusing.

diet consisted of 3 to 3½ servings of low-fat dairy, or 1,200 to 1,600 milligrams of dietary intake from dairy foods, lost 11 per cent of their total body weight. *Most significant, they lost a lot of body fat, especially around the waist area. Dr Zemel concluded that adding three servings of low-fat dairy a day can help you lose up to 70 per cent more weight, increase body fat loss by 64 per cent, and help you lose 47 per cent more belly fat.* Yes, you read that correctly.

I can't tell you how many clients, especially women, complain about not having a flat stomach. Perhaps the most familiar refrain I hear in my practice is, 'I can't get rid of my stomach bulge.'

Most of us do not get enough calcium in our diets. And if you are among those getting the lowest levels of calcium – 255 milligrams a day as opposed to the recommended 800 milligrams for the average adult – you are 84 per cent more likely to be overweight than if you are among those getting the highest level – 1,346 milligrams per day. As Dr Zemel noted in his excellent book, *The Calcium Key*, 'Wouldn't you love to be 84 per cent thinner just by eating more calcium-rich foods every day?'

When calcium levels are not kept optimal, observes Dr Zemel, your body releases a hormone called *calcitriol*, which, in part, *controls* how fat cells work. If you don't get enough calcium in your diet, calcitriol is released and your fat cells get fatter – and you gain more weight! *High-calcium diets suppress calcitriol levels and may speed up weight loss.*

If you're thinking of adding more calcium to your diet, some of you may be wondering if calcium supplements are as efficient at lighting a fuse under excess weight and stored fat as dairy foods. While supplements do help – the subjects in Dr Zemel's study who took an 800-milligram calcium supplement along with 400 to 500 milligrams of dietary calcium daily lost 7.5 per cent of their total weight without reducing calories – they don't provide nearly the same boost as dairy products. 'Dairy products contain a number of bioactive compounds – similar, we believe, to the phytonutrients found in plants – that exert a much stronger effect on fat cells than supplements,' says Dr Zemel. One of these compounds, L-leucine – an essential amino acid – is especially interesting because it helps lower elevated blood-sugar levels and may make fat cells behave more efficiently.

Years ago, I noticed that my clients who added calcium-rich foods to their diet lost more than those who did not. Yogurt is the

Other Points to Keep in Mind

In addition to your weight loss slowing or reaching a plateau, you should also keep the following points in mind regarding your overall health when starting a new weight loss programme.

- **If you have low blood pressure.** If you have low blood pressure, losing weight may cause your pressure to fall further, and you may feel faint (especially if you don't drink enough water or you go too long without eating). When dieting, it's a good idea to drink generous amounts of water, and you may even want to include some higher-salt foods such as pickles and low-calorie soups, to keep your blood pressure stable. In general, if you have a history of low blood pressure, hypoglycaemia, kidney stones, gall bladder problems, low potassium, heart problems, or diabetes, you should lose weight only under the guidance of your doctor.

- **If you change your diet.** In a small number of people, switching from a diet containing a lot of refined carbohydrates to a lower-carbohydrate diet causes a mild 'withdrawal effect'. In the first day or two, they may feel weak or experience headaches. If this happens to you, drink plenty of water and take an aspirin (unless you're allergic to it), and be certain to eat every 3 to 4 hours so your blood sugar stabilizes.

- **If you're taking medications.** If you're taking medications for diabetes, high blood pressure, or other conditions, your prescription may need to be adjusted as you lose weight. Always speak with your doctor or pharmacist if you have any concerns – *never* adjust medication on your own.

- **If you experience leg cramps.** Low potassium or inadequate fluid intake may cause you to experience leg cramps. If you suffer from leg cramps, it's important that you check with your doctor about taking extra potassium. A small banana, two to four slices of cantaloupe, or a glass of tomato juice will help bring your potassium levels back to normal. Your doctor can run a blood test to check your potassium levels. And if you suffer from kidney, gallbladder, or heart disease, you should only diet under the supervision of a doctor.

top calcium-rich food. A 250 g (8 oz) serving of natural yogurt can have up to 490 milligrams – almost half the recommended daily requirement. Other calcium-rich dairy foods include milk (240 ml/8 fl oz has 390) and cottage cheese (60 g/2 oz has 75).

THE 10-DAY TURBOCHARGE DIET

If you're reading these words, you probably have a clear idea about the new standard for weight loss and weight control. You know that

Chef's Miriam's Quick Tips for Preparing Vegetables, Seafood and Meat without Oil or Butter

There are many fast, easy and healthy ways to prepare vegetables, seafood and poultry. The following are a few of Chef Miriam's favourites.

Blanching is a great way to make vegetables. It cooks them enough to take out some of the toughness, but not so much as to take away their crispness and satisfying crunch. Quickly plunge the vegetables into boiling, lightly salted water and cook until they are brightly coloured and still crisp. This way, they will have both crunch and crispness. Often, blanched vegetables are plunged into a bowl of ice water (which stops the cooking). Blanching is a great way to prepare vegetables for a crudité platter. The veggies can be stored in the refrigerator and served to company or eaten as a snack. Drizzle with a touch of seasoned rice vinegar or a good quality balsamic vinaigrette, if you like.

Steaming is a great method for preparing vegetables and seafood. Bring about an inch of water to boil in a medium or large saucepan (depending on the size of your steamer, water shouldn't come in contact with the food). Place the food into a steamer basket. Lower the basket into the saucepan, cover, reduce the heat and steam the food until crisp for vegetables or tender for seafood. Season your food with a splash of lemon juice or good balsamic vinegar, chopped fresh herbs, or sliced spring onions.

Grilling, indoors or out, allows for a crisp exterior and tender interior. For indoor grilling, use a stove-top ridged grill pan (nonstick would be best) and not a frying pan – otherwise, it's not grilling. Prepared spice rubs go well on your unique food history is the 'North Star' to help guide you safely through the world of high-calorie temptations and trigger foods. You're familiar with the strategies for Boxing It In and Boxing It Out. You've learned how to stop using self-defeating 'food baby talk' and replace it with a new script. And you've overcome the feeling that following an eating plan that keeps you trim equals a lifetime of deprivation. You realize that structure gives control. And you know that the goal of this eating plan is not just to lose weight but to permanently change behaviour patterns that have doomed your

meat, seafood and vegetables such as mushrooms and aubergine. You can also season your food with dried herbs such as cumin, oregano, or crushed red-pepper flakes. Or, sprinkle your food with chopped fresh herbs before or after grilling. You can toss sturdy, well-flavoured vegetables such as peppers or onion slices with balsamic or rice vinegar and some herbs (basil) before grilling.

Stir-frying is best done by coating a pan with olive oil cooking spray (don't overcoat) and heating over medium heat for a minute. Add vegetables and a sprinkle of sea salt to get the juices flowing and perhaps even a little dried thyme or rosemary, crumbled in your fingers, for seasoning. Then cook, tossing with two spoons, adding low-fat chicken or vegetable stock, a mixture of

stock and wine (not straight wine, not straight vinegar), or water and wine a tablespoon at a time to keep the vegetables from sticking. A juicy addition would be a chopped fresh tomato or cherry tomatoes. Season with chopped fresh herbs before serving. Very dense vegetables, such as broccoli, carrots and cauliflower should be blanched first or sliced thinly; otherwise, they could scorch before they cook.

Poached vegetables are simmered in a layer of liquid (enough to coat the pan) until cooked. Use chicken stock and water or a mixture of stock and wine, wine and water, or mild vinegar and water. While the poaching liquid is simmering, add some crushed garlic cloves, sliced onion, strips of citrus peel, cracked black pepper, or herb sprigs for flavour before adding your food.

past attempts at dieting. So now that you've absorbed the lessons of the Thin Commandments Diet, you're ready to get started.

Often, when people begin a weight programme, their eating habits have been sloppy and lacked structure and focus. A well-designed, well-organized eating plan – one with clearly defined guidelines, instructions, menus and foods – will help rein in even the most chaotic eaters almost immediately. This is why giving you too many food choices may cause you to feel overwhelmed and lose structure. Once you have your structure firmly entrenched, then you can broaden it.

The menus on pages 220 to 228 give you a list of the possible meal and snack options. You'll find plenty of scrumptious dishes,

How to Avoid 7 Common Kitchen Pitfalls

In many homes, kitchens are more than just a place to eat and prepare food. They're focal points, refuges – places where people meet to discuss their day, socialize, work, watch television, or chat on the telephone. Even the refrigerator has become a shrine of sorts, adorned with magnets, photos, report cards, schedules, favourite aphorisms and reminders about important dates and events.

With so much time spent in the kitchen and its importance in the lives of so many people, the opportunities to overeat are virtually endless. So to avoid problems in the kitchen, follow these seven strategies.

1. **Avoid cooking when you're hungry.** You might end up sampling so much of what you're making that in no time at all, you'll find you've eaten several hundred calories worth of food – before you have even sat down to dinner! If you're concerned, have your 80- to 100-calorie snack before you start cooking or a low-calorie drink.

2. **Don't talk on the telephone or do work in the kitchen.** Doing these things encourages food grazing and mindless eating. Try to limit your 'kitchen conversation' to discussions around the dining-room table. If you have to work, find some place other than your kitchen to do it.

3. **Turn on the lights.** If you come into the kitchen at night, turn on as many lights as you can find (one recent study found that people tend

many of them specially created for you by Chef Miriam – the first female cook at the Four Seasons, one of New York's most celebrated restaurants. I've also included some personal recipes for meals that I serve in my own home.

To know what to eat, simply follow the guidelines provided on the menu. You'll find a list of everything you need to make and prepare your meal selections directly on the menu or in the subsequent recipe section.

As a weight control specialist, I have found that for most people, the best choice for breakfast during the diet is a protein – especially a high-calcium or light choice such as the Omelette Supreme (page 220), Savoury Smoked Salmon (page 220), or Fruit and Yogurt Bliss

to eat more in dimly lit rooms).

4. **Don't go into the kitchen when you're upset.** People sometimes eat when they're anxious, nervous, or distressed.

5. **Avoid eating while reading and watching TV.** Pleasurable activities such as reading and watching television can cause you to lose track of the amounts you're eating since your mind is often absorbed in what you're doing. Even worse, you may find yourself eating until your programme is over, or you've finished reading. Sitting next to the food makes it too easy to eat extra and keeps food before your eyes all the time.

6. **Don't become the 'garbage bin'.** It's not your job to finish everyone's leftovers. If you're in the habit of picking or nibbling at what remains on other people's plates, have a piece of gum or a Listerine Breath Strip to help keep you away from the scraps. Always keep the Listerine Breath Strips or a Halls Sugar-Free cough drop on your kitchen worktop.

7. **Beware of the kitchen worktop.** *Don't forget that in your house, the single most dangerous spot in terms of food control is the kitchen worktop.* I've found that people invariably pick or nibble on anything that's lying around – even if they're not hungry. A good rule of thumb is to keep your surfaces free of temptation, especially in the form of nibble or finger foods.

(page 221). A protein-based breakfast takes longer to digest than a breakfast without any protein and is likely to keep you satisfied for several hours. I also like a protein breakfast because it will get you out of the habit of eating too many bad carbohydrates, such as croissants, bagels, white bread, or low-fibre breakfast cereals early in the day. There's growing evidence that such a breakfast may impair your body's ability to keep blood-sugar levels stable as the day wears on. In other words, your hunger increases even if you have a protein for lunch or dinner.

For the most part, the breakfast choices on the 10-Day Turbo-Charge Diet are quick and easy to make. However, if you're running to an appointment or have an early meeting at work, you can select one of the 'On the Go' choices such as Cheese Melt on GG Scandinavian Bran Crispbread (page 220). If, however, you select the Atkins' Morning Shine Bar, be aware that while this choice contains protein, people who abuse confectionery may find that a similar pattern emerges with bars. If this is your history, this item is not the best choice. Instead, consider the GG 'n' Egg or Ham 'n' Cheese Breakfast Sandwich, both of which you can prepare in less than 5 minutes in your microwave.

In making your selections for lunch and dinner, the best choices for rapid weight loss are the seafood and green vegetable meals. You can try the Cucumber Prawn Salad (page 222), or Chef Miriam's Grilled Salmon Salad (page 234). If you don't care for fish, try the Ham 'n' Cheese Breakfast Sandwich (page 220), Chef Miriam's Many Vegetable Omelette (page 220), or my recipe for Cold Meat Rolls (page 224).

When you peruse the lunch and dinner choices, you may notice that I often recommend bran crackers, especially the GG Scandinavian Bran Crispbread, in lieu of bread. There are many reasons for this. Bran crackers serve the same purpose as bread, give crunch without the calories, offer more nutrition for far fewer calories, provide more fibre and volume than wholegrain bread, and for people who have a history of abusing bread products, they avoid the association of bread with meals. You may even discover, as have many of my clients, that you do not want to return to bread products. However, if you find that you still want bread, one piece of light or wheat bread (45 calories or less a slice) once or twice a week is allowed. Truth be told, my goal is really to wean you off bread since the overconsumption of bread and bread products is one of the biggest reasons why people fail on diets. I often joke with my clients that if not for the baker's oven, their great figures wouldn't have gone up in smoke!

If you decide to eat out, don't order any of the items that appear on the menu unless you know exactly how they're prepared. For example, restaurant versions of tuna or chicken salad may contain loads of high-fat mayonnaise or high-calorie dressing. The word 'salad' in the title of a menu item is no guarantee that it'll be low in calories. Once again, ask yourself (or your server) what the salad comes with and how it is prepared.

If you find a food that comes in either water or oil, such as tuna or certain canned vegetables, always select the one that comes in water. As a general rule, oil should be limited to cooking sprays. If you must have oil with your meal, limit it to 1 or 2 teaspoons of olive or rapeseed (canola) oil on a salad or one of the recommended vegetables, *and do not use it as part of your overall food preparation.* Many of my clients who like oil find that 1 or 2 teaspoons of truffle oil goes a lot further than other oils they've tried.

Although I don't insist, it's best to avoid alcohol completely during the 10-day diet, unless it's for a special event. In that case, most of my clients find that the best choice is a small (90-ml/3-fl oz) glass of dry red or white wine, scotch or vodka with water, soda water or diet tonic water. Don't drink on an empty stomach – and order a second, non-alcoholic drink, and alternate drinking that with the alcoholic drink.

How about fruit? The sweet taste of most fruits comes from the sugar in the fruit. Fruit sugar will not raise your blood sugar as much as table sugar and the fibre in the skin of fruits such as apples and pears may help slow down absorption (the fibre delays your stomach's ability to get to the sugar). Since I want you to get the benefits of fruit (fibre, vitamins, minerals), I've included a limited number in the 10-Day TurboCharge Diet that don't have a lot of calories and won't cause too many problems with your blood sugar, such as grapefruit, cantaloupe, apples and strawberries. If you're a sugar-sensitive person, it's best to have it as part of a meal or as a snack that includes protein. Some of my clients who fall into the sugar-sensitive category will take half the recommended amount of fruit and combine it with a low-fat protein such as a wedge of

Laughing Cow Light cheese. And be sure to eat the protein first to help control your blood sugar.

It's also a good idea to avoid fruit juices, which are frequently loaded with sugar, provide little or no fibre (except for fresh-squeezed orange juice), and can raise your blood sugar as much as a fizzy drink or chocolate bar. The only exception to this rule would be tomato juice or V8 Vegetable Juice, because I've found they act as appetite suppressants.

While this eating plan is geared for 10 days, often my clients will ask when's the best time to introduce a greater variety of foods. My answer is twofold. You can do this once you've lost 2.25–4.5 kg (5–10 lb). Or, you can delay widening the diet if you lose weight slowly or have lost weight slowly in the past. Others may elect to stay on the 10-day diet for longer because they feel comfortable with its structure and are not ready to eat an increased variety of foods, particularly more caloric ones.

For health purposes, it's not recommended that you lose more than 1 kg (2 lb) a week after the first 14 days. Since the diet is such a powerful plan for weight loss, some people will still be losing more than 1 kg (2 lb) after the first 2 weeks. If this applies to you, it's best to add an extra fruit, a few more servings of GG & Cheese, or eat more chicken in lieu of the fruit to slow down the loss.

Always have a complete physical before going on this diet.

The 10-Day TurboCharge Diet

The core of my 10-Day TurboCharge Diet is eggs, fish and high-calcium dairy foods such as yogurt and low-fat cheese, along with my recommended high-fibre crispbread. Many other selections are given for those who prefer other types of meals or who may need a little more variety. I cannot emphasize enough, however, that for the optimal benefit, the core foods should be selected. For each meal, an asterisk (*) will be placed against the selections that will produce the accelerated weight loss. Whatever meal you do select, you should experience significant weight loss with the 10-Day TurboCharge Diet. Enjoy!

Note on suggested serving size: When two amounts are indicated, the lower amount applies to women and the higher amount to men.

Note on high-fibre crackers: My first choice is the GG Scandinavian Bran Crispbread, since it is the only thick cracker with a mere 18 calories, 3 grams of appetite-quenching fibre, and 3 grams of carbohydrates (0 net carbs!) If you are waiting for a shipment to arrive at your local health food shop, you may *temporarily* substitute any other thick high-fibre cracker that has no more than 30 calories and at least 1.5 grams of fibre. All crackers that I have come across have more calories and carbohydrates and less fibre than the GGs, so I strongly recommend you only use the GGs.

Note on light cheese: My top choice of a light cheese is Laughing Cow Light, since it comes premeasured in individually wrapped triangles (each of which is only 25 calories). If you can't find Laughing Cow Light, temporarily use the Laughing Cow, which are 22 more calories, until you find a source of the light ones, or use 2 tablespoons of Quark soft cheese or WeightWatchers soft cheese for each Laughing Cow Light. But I strongly recommend Laughing Cow Light because it is low in calories, it is contained in a small package so you're less likely to be tempted to have more, and it is instantly spreadable. Remember: Laughing Cow is wrapped and can travel with you anywhere.

--- **Breakfast Menu** ---

Quick and Easy Breakfast

These items may be enjoyed every day and take less than 15 minutes to prepare.

*Omelette Supreme

Prepare with either 4 egg whites, 1 yolk and 3 egg whites, or 170 g (6 oz) of egg substitute, and 1 tablespoon of Parmesan cheese. If you like, you may have 1 or 2 GG Scandinavian Bran Crispbreads or comparable high-fibre crackers with your meal. Prepare with olive oil cooking spray.

*Ham 'n' Eggs

Prepare in the same way as the Omelette Supreme, and add 1 slice of any 20- to 25-calorie light ham in lieu of cheese.

Cheese Melt on GG Crispbread

Melt 1 or 2 pieces of low-fat cheese (1 or 2 Laughing Cow Light wedges) on 2 to 4 GG Scandinavian Bran Crispbreads or similar high-fibre crackers.

Apple Cottage-Cheese Delight

115–230 g (4–8 oz) low-fat or cottage cheese on GG Scandinavian Bran Crispbread, topped with a teaspoon of apple sauce, or a thin slice of apple, and sprinkled with cinnamon.

*Top Choice for accelerated weight loss

Gourmet Breakfast

These special choices may be enjoyed one to three times per week, especially on weekends.

Bacon 'n' Eggs

Prepare with either 4 egg whites, 1 yolk and 3 egg whites, or 170 g (6 oz) of egg substitute. Or, have 2 hardboiled eggs. If you have scrambled eggs, add 115 g (4 oz) of mushrooms and broccoli and a slice of onion. Serve with 1 thin slice of grilled back bacon (trimmed of fat).

Savoury Smoked Salmon

Use 60–90 g (2–3 oz) of smoked salmon on 2 or 3 GG or other high-fibre crackers with a thick layer of Quark soft cheese, which is virtually fat-free, or a thin layer of a low-fat garlic-flavoured cheese spread.

On-the-Go Breakfast

Try these delicious options when you're on the go or don't have time for a sit-down meal.

Ham 'n' Cheese Breakfast Sandwich

Follow the recipe for the cheese melt but add 1 or 2 slices of any light ham that has 20–25 calories a slice).

Fruit and Yogurt Bliss

Take 170–230 g (6–8 oz) of fat-free or light yogurt and if desired sweeten with Splenda, ½ teaspoon of cinnamon and 1 tablespoon of low-carb fruit preserves. For crunch, add 1 tablespoon of bran cereal. You may also add 3 or 4 sliced strawberries or 3 or 4 small cubes of cantaloupe to the yogurt.

Hard-Boiled Eggs

1 or 2 hard-boiled eggs or 170 g (6 oz) of egg substitute on 2 GG crackers or similar crackers.

Sweet Shake

One low-cal protein shake made with skimmed milk. For added flavour, you may add a few sliced strawberries and ½ teaspoon of cinnamon.

Atkins Morning Shine Breakfast Bar

Comes in a number of different flavours, and each bar contains 135 to 145 calories.

Lunch Menu

Quick and Easy Lunch

These items may be enjoyed every day.

Yogurt Jubilee

Combine 340 g (12 oz) plain, fat-free yogurt (Fage Total Yogurt) or light yogurt with 4 tablespoons of dried onion soup mix, plus dill and spices, and serve as a dip with a tray of cut-up vegetables or a plate of steamed green and white vegetables and/or a salad with nonfat dressing or a flavoured balsamic vinaigrette. (For hunger control, yogurt must be combined with vegetables.)

Ham and Cheese Sandwich

Melt 1 or 2 triangles of Laughing Cow Light (or similar cheese) over 4 slices of light ham (20–25 calories a slice) on 4 GG or comparable high-fibre crackers. Do not use regular cheese.

Lightning-Fast Fish

1 or 2 grilled white fish fillets, sprinkled with lemon juice, cayenne and oregano and served on a bed of spinach or steamed green and white vegetables (see page 212).

Smoked Salmon Salad

Put 2 or 3 pieces of smoked salmon on a tossed salad and add some capers.

*Good Ol' Franks

2 to 3 low-fat franks (75 calories or less per frank – you'll usually find the lower calorie ones in jars rather than at the deli counter) on a bed of sauerkraut or spinach with steamed low-carb green and white vegetables and/or a salad with nonfat dressing or a flavoured balsamic vinaigrette. (Try grilling the franks on the George Foreman Grill.)

GG Sandwich with Turkey and Cheddar

Prepare this delicious sandwich with 2 or 3 slices of light turkey breast meat, a slice of low-fat cheddar cheese and 4 GG crackers. Add a thin layer of spicy mustard. Enjoy with a plateful of steamed green and white vegetables.

GGs with Cheese and Fruit

Mix 60 g (2 oz) Quark soft cheese with 2 tablespoons chopped strawberries, 2 tablespoons blueberries and a pinch of cinnamon. Spread on 3 GG crackers.

Dilled Egg Salad

See recipe, page 237.

*Many Vegetable Omelette

Made with 4 egg whites, or 1 yolk and 3 egg whites, or 170 g (6 oz) of egg substitute and 1 slice of light cheese (such as Laughing Cow Light), or 1 tablespoon of Parmesan cheese. If you like, you may have 1 or 2 bran crackers with your meal. Prepare with olive oil cooking spray or use a coated pan without oil. Enjoy with a plateful of steamed green and white vegetables.

*Cucumber Prawn Salad

Mix 145–170 g (5–6 oz) of cooked prawns with 1 tablespoon of Hellman's Light Mayonnaise. Add chopped celery, a little chopped onion, tomato and garlic powder, and serve on slivers of cucumber or over a mixed green salad.

Apple Cottage-Cheese Delight

Feel free to enjoy this breakfast choice for lunch (just add 25 per cent more cottage cheese) on 4 GGs or other bran crackers, and top with ½ to 1 teaspoon cinnamon.

Grilled Salmon Salad

See recipe, page 234. Those eating out may have grilled fish or prawns with a salad or steamed vegetables. Make sure the fish is grilled dry, with no added butter or oil.

*Top Choice for accelerated weight loss

Gourmet Lunch

These special choices are to be used 1 or 2 times per week, especially on weekends.

Turkey or Chicken Salad

Mix 60–115 g (2–4 oz) of white meat chicken or turkey with a tossed salad. You may add 1 tablespoon of vinaigrette, 1 tablespoon of grated Parmesan cheese, or 1 or 2 slices of Laughing Cow Light, 4 Spanish olives and 3 or 4 slivers of sun-dried tomato (packed in water).

General G's Chinese Seafood

For best results, sauté or steam 115–170 g (4–6 oz) of seafood, such as prawns or scallops in rice wine or stock with spring onions, ginger and garlic. *The seafood should not be sautéed in oil!* Serve with steamed Chinese vegetables prepared in the same way. For added flavour, try a little light soy sauce, or serve in a bowl with wonton soup (minus the wonton noodles). The same recipe may be prepared with white meat chicken, but it's not a first choice for accelerated weight loss.

Dr G's Light Pizza

Spray a baking sheet with olive oil cooking spray. Top 3 or 4 GG crackers with a sprinkle of low-fat grated cheese, a little low-fat Napoletana sauce, mushrooms, garlic and oregano. Bake until cheese melts.

Totally Tofu

Prepare the Chinese-themed dish (General G's Chinese) with 60–115 g (2–4 oz) of tofu and mixed steamed vegetables.

Mustard-Crumbed Chicken

Mix 1 tablespoon grainy mustard with 1 tablespoon fat-free natural yogurt, add a 115 g/4 oz skinless chicken breast and turn it to coat both sides. Finely crush 3 GG bran crackers and roll the chicken in the crumbs. Spray with some olive oil cooking spray and bake in a 190°C/375°F/gas 5 oven until the chicken is no longer pink in the middle – about 15–17 minutes.

Portobello Sandwich

Grill 1 low-cal veggie burger and serve over slivers of portobello mushrooms topped with alfalfa sprouts. For added zest, try a little fat-free BBQ sauce. Enjoy with a salad and/or a plateful of steamed green and white vegetables.

Hearty Seafood Broth

455–685 g (1–1½ lb) of mussels cooked in wine and stock with mushrooms and garlic (no oil, butter or tomato sauce).

Many Vegetable Soup

See recipe, page 232.

*Pink Tuscan Tuna

Make this delicious salad with 115–170 g (4–6 oz) of water-packed light tuna (which is low in mercury). Mix in a food processor with 1 table-spoon of Hellman's Light Mayonnaise and 1 red pimento pepper (water-packed only). After it's mixed, sprinkle on 1 teaspoon of crushed garlic or chopped onion and 2 tablespoons chopped tomato. Place over a tossed salad or uncooked spinach, and top with chives, 1 tablespoon of grated Parmesan cheese, and 1 tablespoon of cut-up sun-dried tomato (not packed in oil).

Leaning Vegetable Stacks

See recipe, page 236.

Better than Deli Tuna Salad

See recipe, page 233.

On-the-Go Lunch

Try these delicious choices when you're on the go or don't have time for a sit-down meal.

GG Veggie-Cheese Crunch

Takes only 4 minutes to prepare. Mix 60 g (2 oz) Quark soft cheese with some chopped cucumber, 2 tablespoons chopped red or green pepper and a tablespoon thinly sliced spring onion. Season to taste, spread evenly over 3 GG crispbreads and top with some chopped tomato.

2 Sweet Shakes

Double the breakfast amount.

Fast-Food Lunch

Heavenly Roll

8 to 10 pieces of sashimi or cucumber sashimi (fish rolled in cucumber skin). Serve with wasabi mustard and a light soy sauce. Add a bowl of miso soup (it's high in sodium, so don't weigh yourself for 24 hours).

Cold Meat Rolls

Start with large lettuce leaves. Place 4–6 slices of light cold meat on the leaves, and roll around cucumber or courgette sticks.

*Top Choice for accelerated weight loss

Dinner Menu

Quick and Easy Dinner

These items may be enjoyed every day. If you prefer, any lunch main course may be enjoyed in lieu of dinner.

Frozen Low-Carb Dinners

Select any frozen ready-meal (such as Weight Watchers) that's low-carb and contains no more than 300 calories. Pick the new low-carb main courses where rice, potatoes and pastas have been replaced with lower-carb vegetables. Have a big salad and steamed green and white vegetables.

Chicken Parmesan

Start with 115–170 g (4–6 oz) skinless cooked chicken breasts. Spray a baking sheet with olive oil cooking spray. Cut each breast in two crosswise and top each piece with 2–3 tablespoons low-fat tomato sauce and 1 tablespoon grated Parmesan, crushed garlic and a little parsley. Preheat your oven to 180°C/350°F/gas 4, and heat briefly until the cheese melts. Serve with steamed vegetables and a salad with fat-free dressing or flavoured balsamic vinaigrette

Grilled Fish or Seafood

Prepare with 115–170 g (4–6 oz) of white fish or seafood such as prawns or crab meat. Serve with steamed vegetables and a tossed salad.

Scallop and Vegetable Packets

See recipe, page 252.

Dr G's World Famous Courgette/Aubergine Parmigiana

See recipe, page 238. Women may eat ½ to ⅔ of the recipe. Men can eat ⅔ or the entire recipe (it's high in sodium).

Delicious Veggie Burgers

Prepare two low-cal veggie burgers (use burgers that are less than 130 calories) and serve on a bed of spinach with some steamed vegetables or a bowl of my recommended soups. For added flavour, top with a tablespoon of fat-free BBQ sauce.

Good Ol' Franks

Increase the lunch menu to 3 or 4 franks.

Dr G's Chef's Salad Light

Make with 90–145 g (3–5 oz) of sliced fresh turkey, 1 slice of light Swiss cheese, or other nutty cheese such as Leerdammer Light (not more than 80 calories a slice), and 1 or 2 slices of light ham (no more than 25 calories a slice). For a dressing, try balsamic vinegar mixed with lemon and mustard. Have with green and white vegetables.

Gourmet Dinner

These items may be enjoyed every day.

Creole Crumbed Prawns
See recipe, page 241.

Sticks of Fish
Prepare simply with 3 or 4 frozen fish sticks (or fingers) – 'healthy choice' if available. Serve with 300 g (10½ oz) of steamed asparagus and 1 tablespoon of low-cal dressing.

Fish 'n' Chips
Made with Sticks of Fish (see above) and Oven 'Fried' Courgette chips (see recipe, page 235)

Dr G's Prawn Scampi
Start by sautéing 170–230 g (6–8 oz) of prawns in a pan coated with 1 or 2 sprays of olive oil spray. Add 2 or 3 tablespoons of crushed garlic with a little wine and a sprinkle of parsley for added flavour.

Mussels with Soy and Sherry
See recipe, page 251.

Roasted Sage-Lemon Salmon
See recipe, page 249.

Seafood in Brodo
See recipe, page 248.

Chef Miriam's Dinners

Yucatan-Style Grilled Swordfish
Note: Swordfish is high in mercury and should not be consumed more than 1 or 2 times a week maximum, and not at all by pregnant or nursing women.
See recipe, page 254.

Oven-Steamed Salmon Hong Kong-Style
See recipe, page 246.

Seafood Salad Positano
See recipe, page 250.

Top Choice for accelerated weight loss

Snacks and Mini-meals

Women should have a maximum of two snacks or mini-meals per day. Men may have up to three. One of those snacks or mini-meals is required in the critical late afternoon to early evening period of 3 to 5 p.m. Others may be enjoyed midmorning, in the evening, or right before dinner to prevent any hunger. Or you may elect to omit the additional snack(s) and use your 'free foods' instead. The critical determinant is that you should avoid being hungry at any time during the day.

Where two amounts are indicated, women should have the lower amount and men the larger amount.

Yogurt: Fage Total Yogurt 0% or comparable fat-free yogurt

Total Yogurt is around 80 calories; adjust the other yogurt to get between 80 and 100 calories per serving.

V-8 Juice or a low-sodium vegetable or tomato juice, 180 ml (6 fl oz) serving

Grapefruit

3 halves = 1 snack. If you select this snack, you should have half a grapefruit with each meal. Since this is a snack designed to be a calorie-budget stretcher, it works best in that capacity immediately after a meal. Women should avoid a large grapefruit. (Do not have more than 3 halves of grapefruit per day.)

Bowl of Soup

A serving of one of the many less-than-1%-fat tinned soups, or the portable envelopes of dried soups that have 70 to 80 calories – may be enjoyed with 1 high-fibre cracker (not more than 30 calories).

Cheese Omelette

2 egg whites and 1 tablespoon of Parmesan cheese mixed with cut-up low-carb, green and white vegetables. You may omit the cheese.

Dr G's Light Pizza

See recipe, page 223. Women may have 2 cracker pizzas and men may have up to 3.

Hot Dogs

1 or 2 light hot dogs (the tinned variety are often less than 50 calories each) on a bed of sauerkraut or steamed low-carb green and white vegetables.

Dr G's BLT

2 GG Scandinavian Bran Crispbreads or comparable high-fibre cracker, lettuce, a thin slice of tomato, 1 slice of ready-to-eat cooked back bacon (trimmed of any fat) and a thin spread of extra-light mayonnaise.

2 Laughing Cow Cheese Wedges

Yogurt Crunch 'n' Berry

170 g (6 oz) of Total 0% Yogurt or comparable (85 calories or less per serving) yogurt sprinkled with 2 teaspoons of All-Bran cereal, one sliced medium-size strawberry, and Splenda.

Cappuccino with Skimmed Milk (240-ml/8-fl oz serving)

If you would like a sweet accompaniment, try one of the high-fibre crackers and a teaspoon of reduced-sugar or low-carb fruit preserves.

Virtually Fat-Free Cottage Cheese (115–170g/4–6 oz)

You can mix cottage cheese and 1 tablespoon of low-carb fruit preserves.

Crackers 'n' Cold Meat Sandwich

2 GG Scandinavian Bran Crispbreads or comparable high-fibre cracker with 2 or 3 slices of any light cold meat (20 to 25 calories per slice) topped with mustard or a thin spread of extra-light mayonnaise (optional: lettuce and a thin slice of tomato).

Prawn Cocktail

4 to 6 medium-size prawns topped with 1 tablespoon extra-light crème fraîche mixed with a little tomato purée and a dash of Tabasco.

One Hard-Boiled Egg

You can chop the egg over a green salad, or you can use 115 g (4 oz) of egg substitute (preferably with cut-up vegetables or salad).

Top Choice for accelerated weight loss

Free Foods

The following foods are unlimited unless otherwise indicated:

- Coffee
- Tea
- Tomato juice (120 ml/4 fl oz); 1 to 2 times per day; preferably low salt)
- Diet soft drinks
- All condiments
- Green and white low-calorie, low-carb vegetables (see page 205). This does not include peas, onions, the squash family, potatoes, avocado, and obviously tomatoes, carrots, beans, chickpeas and lentils.
- Diet Hot Chocolate (Do not buy any hot chocolate with more than 35 calories.) You can have a maximum of two of these per day.

The following foods are free if used as indicated, with the lower amount for women and the higher amount for men:

- 2 egg whites per day (may be combined with free green and white vegetables to make an omelette or vegetable soufflé)
- ½ grapefruit a day (eaten with your heaviest caloric meal of the day)
- 2 GG crackers or one high-fibre, low-carb substitute cracker
- Sugar-free jelly.
- 1 sugar-free gum. Have no more than 3 or 4 pieces per day.
- 240 ml (8 fl oz) of fat-free, low-salt chicken stock (may be combined with the green and white vegetables such as spinach or cabbage to make a free vegetable soup). You can even add one of your free egg whites to the boiling soup to make an instant egg-drop soup, or add cooked, drained spinach to have an Italian spinach soup (Stracchiatella).

Amazing Lemony Soup with Crab and Vegetables

Prep: 5 minutes ● Cook: 9 minutes

This soup is amazing because it's so easy, so delicious and so low in calories. Cooked chopped chicken could be used instead of the crab.

> 400 ml (14 fl oz) fat-free reduced-sodium chicken stock
> 1 garlic clove, peeled and cut in half
> 100 g (3½ oz) sliced mushrooms (use pre-sliced)
> 75 g (2½ oz) thinly sliced courgette
> 50 g (1¾ oz) baby spinach
> 60 g (2 oz) crab meat, picked over
> ¼ teaspoon grated lemon zest
> 1 tablespoon fresh lemon juice

In a medium saucepan, combine the stock and garlic. Cover and bring to the boil over high heat. Add the mushrooms and courgette; reduce the heat to medium, cover and simmer until the vegetables are tender, about 3 minutes.

Stir in the spinach and cook just until wilted, about 30 seconds. Remove from the heat and stir in the crab, lemon zest and juice. Discard the garlic. Serve immediately.

Makes 1 serving (540 ml/19 fl oz)

Per serving: 130 calories, 4 g fat, 1 g saturated fat, 18 g protein, 4 g carbohydrates, 3 g dietary fibre, 607 mg sodium

Dilled Cucumber and Yogurt Soup

Prep: 10 minutes

This soup is very refreshing on a warm day – best yet, no cooking is necessary. Sip from a mug and accompany with a GG Scandinavian Bran Crispbread.

100 g (3½ oz) sliced cucumber

2 tablespoons chopped sweet onion

1 tablespoon snipped fresh dill

1 teaspoon rice wine vinegar

½ small garlic clove

¼ teaspoon dried mint, crumbled

⅛ teaspoon salt

170 g (6 oz) natural fat-free yogurt

Freshly ground black pepper, to taste

Put the cucumber, onion, dill, vinegar, garlic, mint and salt in a food processor and process until very finely chopped.

Add the yogurt and process until smooth. Season to taste with pepper. Serve immediately, with a slice of cucumber floating on top, or cover and chill until ready to serve.

Makes 1 serving (360 ml/12 fl oz)

Per serving: 155 calories, 2 g fat, 1 g saturated fat, 12 g protein, 23 g carbohydrates, 3 g dietary fibre, 547 mg sodium

Many Vegetable Soup

Prep: 15 minutes ● Cook: 23 minutes

You'll want to keep this soup on hand for lunches and snacks. If you like, add a little protein to each bowl with some chopped hard-boiled egg white or a tablespoon of grated Parmesan or shredded light mozzarella.

1.2 litres (40 fl oz) fat-free reduced-sodium chicken stock

100 g (3½ oz) thinly sliced celery, with some leaves

1 small onion, halved and thinly sliced

1 garlic clove, crushed

2 teaspoons chopped fresh thyme leaves

230 g (8 oz) thinly sliced cauliflower florets

150 g (5½ oz) cut green beans, 1 cm (½ in) pieces

230 g (8 oz) diagonally sliced asparagus

230 g (8 oz) thinly sliced yellow summer squash or courgette

¼ teaspoon salt

In a large saucepan, combine the stock, celery, onion, garlic and thyme. Cover and bring to a boil over high heat.

Stir in the cauliflower and green beans. Reduce the heat to medium, cover, and simmer until crisp-tender, 5 minutes. Stir in the asparagus, squash and salt. Cover and simmer until the vegetables are tender, about 5 minutes longer. Serve hot.

Makes 4 servings (1.2 litres/3½ pints)

Per serving: 70 calories, 2 g fat, 0.5 g saturated fat, 6 g protein, 8 g carbohydrates, 4 g dietary fibre, 224 mg sodium

Better Than Deli Tuna Salad

Prep: 10 minutes

Fresher, leaner and full of crunch – you'll never need deli tuna salad after enjoying this slimmed-down version. Serve on a bed of crisp mixed greens spritzed with lemon juice or balsamic vinegar, or spread the salad on GG Scandinavian Bran Crispbreads.

> **90 g (3 oz) water-packed tuna, drained and flaked**
>
> **1 hard-boiled egg white, chopped**
>
> **45 g (1½ oz) each finely chopped red and green peppers**
>
> **30 g (1 oz) chopped celery**
>
> **2–3 tablespoons chopped dill pickle**
>
> **1½ tablespoons light mayonnaise**
>
> **1 tablespoon chopped red onion**
>
> **Salt and freshly ground pepper to taste**

In a salad bowl, combine all ingredients and stir with a fork to blend well. Serve immediately, or cover and refrigerate until ready to serve.

Makes 1 serving

Per serving: 230 calories, 10 g fat, 2 g saturated fat, 23 g protein, 7 g carbohydrates, 2 g dietary fibre, 853 mg sodium

Grilled Salmon Salad

Prep: 6 minutes ● Cook: 14 minutes ● Cooling time: 10 minutes

Fresh is best but a 100 g (3½ oz) can of salmon can be used in a pinch. Don't discard the tiny soft bones from the canned salmon; they're full of calcium. Serve this salad on a bed of mixed greens, with vegetable sticks or GG Scandinavian Bran Crispbreads. (*Note:* You can substitute another type of fish for the salmon if you desire.)

One 90–115 g (3–4 oz) skinned salmon fillet
⅛ teaspoon coarsely ground black pepper
Pinch salt
1 hard-boiled egg white, chopped
30 g (1 oz) chopped cucumber
45 g (1½ oz) chopped yellow, orange or red pepper
1 spring onion, thinly sliced
1 tablespoon coarsely chopped pimento-stuffed green olives
1 tablespoon extra-light mayonnaise
1 teaspoon grainy mustard

Coat a small nonstick frying pan with olive oil cooking spray. Heat over medium heat for 2 minutes.

Season the salmon with pepper and salt. Place in the frying pan and cook until lightly browned on the outside and just opaque in the thickest part, 2–4 minutes per side. Transfer to a plate and let stand 10 minutes to cool.

Break the salmon into coarse flakes. Put in a salad bowl and mix in the egg white, cucumber, pepper, spring onion, olives, mayonnaise and mustard. Serve immediately, or cover and refrigerate until ready to serve.

Makes 1 serving

Per serving: 270 calories, 14 g fat, 2.5 g saturated fat, 27 g protein, 8 g carbohydrates, 2 g dietary fibre, 690 mg sodium

Oven 'Fried' Courgette

Prep: 5 minutes ● Cook: 20 minutes

There are two ways to do this: you can sliver the courgette in a food processor fitted with the slicing blade, and you'll get very thin 'chips'. Some will bake up crisp; some will be meltingly soft. Or you can make thin wedges, which will be a touch crispy on the outside and tender on the inside. Both are good. And both need to be eaten hot from the oven.

> **2 medium courgettes (about 455 g/1 lb), trimmed and cut into**
> **wedges 5 mm (¼ in) wide and 10 cm (4 in) long, or halved**
> **lengthwise (to fit in the food processor's feed tube)**
> **3 large egg whites**
> **¼ teaspoon salt**

Preheat the oven to 260°C/500°F/highest gas setting. If making wedges, coat a large heavy baking sheet with olive oil cooking spray; if making slivers, you'll need to prepare 2 baking sheets.

In a large bowl, whisk the egg whites and salt until frothy. Add the courgette and toss to coat well; let stand for 5 minutes.

Arrange the courgette wedges in single layers with a cut side down on the prepared baking sheet, letting the excess egg white drip into the bowl. Arrange the slivers in single layers on the 2 sheets, without worrying if some overlap. Mist the courgette with olive oil cooking spray.

Bake the wedges, turning once to the other cut side, until golden, about 15 minutes. Bake the slivers without turning, moving the pans to the opposite racks halfway though baking, until lightly browned in spots, about 12 minutes.

Let courgette stand on the baking sheet(s) for a minute after removing from the oven. Scrape onto a plate and serve hot.

Makes 2 servings

Per serving: 60 calories, 1 g fat, 0 g saturated fat, 8 g protein, 8 g carbohydrates, 2 g dietary fibre, 280 mg sodium

Leaning Vegetable Stacks

Prep: 15 minutes ● Cook: 37 minutes

Your diet-conscious friends and family will love this satisfying dish. These stacks lean slightly, not unlike the Tower of Pisa.

> **3 large garlic cloves, crushed**
>
> **2 tablespoons chopped fresh rosemary**
>
> **1 tablespoon chopped fresh oregano**
>
> **$\frac{1}{2}$ teaspoon freshly ground black pepper**
>
> **$\frac{1}{4}$ teaspoon salt**
>
> **4 medium portabello mushroom caps (10 cm/4 in), wiped clean, stems cut out**
>
> **Four 1 cm ($\frac{1}{2}$-in) slices peeled aubergine, cut crosswise**
>
> **1 large red pepper, cut into thin strips**
>
> **2 medium tomatoes, each cored and cut in 4 slices**
>
> **170 g (6 oz) Quark soft cheese**
>
> **125 g (4$\frac{1}{2}$ oz) light mozzarella cheese, grated**

Preheat the grill. Coat 2 rimmed baking sheets with olive oil cooking spray.

In a cup, mix the garlic, rosemary, oregano, pepper and salt.

On one of the baking sheets, place the mushrooms and aubergine. Mist with olive oil cooking spray and sprinkle with some of the herb mixture. Turn the vegetables over and repeat.

Place the pepper strips in a small bowl and toss with some herb mixture. Arrange the tomatoes on the other prepared baking sheet; sprinkle the remaining herb mixture on both sides.

Grill the mushrooms and aubergine 8–13 cm (3–5 in) from the heat until lightly browned, about 5 minutes. Turn and grill 5 minutes longer, until the aubergine is tender (mushrooms won't be done). Transfer the aubergine to a plate.

Place the pepper on the sheet next to the mushrooms. Grill, turning mushrooms and pepper often, until tender, 4–6 minutes. Remove from the heat.

Grill the tomatoes without turning, until heated through, about 5 minutes. Remove from the heat. Turn the oven to 220°C/425°F/gas 7.

Prepare the stacks like this: on a baking sheet, place the mushrooms open side up. Fill each with 3 tablespoons quark. Arrange an aubergine slice and 2 tomato slices overlapping slightly on the mushrooms. Sprinkle with the pepper strips and mozzarella. Bake until hot and the cheese has melted, 4–6 minutes. Serve immediately.

Makes 4 servings

Per serving: 130 calories, 5 g fat, 2 g saturated fat, 14 g protein, 8 g carbohydrates, 3 g dietary fibre, 300 mg sodium

Dilled Egg Salad

Prep: 12 minutes

If you don't care for dill, add parsley or a pinch of a dried herb you like. Serve with GG Scandinavian Bran Crispbreads and/or steamed broccoli. Add a fruit that's allowed and you have an entire meal.

> 1 hard-boiled egg, chopped (can use just the white), plus 3 hard-boiled egg whites, chopped
> 30 g (1 oz) finely chopped celery
> 2 tablespoons chopped sweet white onion
> 2 tablespoons snipped fresh dill
> 2 tablespoons extra-light mayonnaise
> 1 tablespoon chopped fresh tomato
> ½ teaspoon Dijon mustard
> ⅛ teaspoon each salt and freshly ground black pepper

In a salad bowl, combine all ingredients and stir with a fork to blend well. Serve immediately or cover and refrigerate until ready to serve.

Makes 1 serving

Per serving: 170 calories, 6 g fat, 2 g saturated fat, 18 g protein, 9 g carbohydrates, 1 g dietary fibre, 810 mg sodium

Dr G's World Famous Low-Calorie Courgette/Aubergine Parmigiana

Prep: 12 minutes ● Cook: 37 minutes

While dining on this festive fare, I suggest serving a crisp green salad tossed with low-fat vinaigrette. If you like, add 145 g (5 oz) sliced white button mushrooms that have been sautéed in a nonstick pan with 1 tablespoon white wine. To make the meal truly memorable, play some Italian music in the background – an opera by Verdi would be most appropriate.

See the Dining for One version opposite.

> 2 teaspoons dried Italian herb seasoning
> ¼ teaspoon salt
> ¼ teaspoon crushed red pepper flakes
> ¼ teaspoon garlic powder
> 1 medium aubergine (about 455 g/1 lb), peeled and cut lengthwise into 1-cm (½-in) slices
> 2 medium courgettes (about 455 g/1 lb), cut lengthwise into 1-cm (½-in) slices
> 240 ml (8 fl oz) fat-free or low-fat marinara sauce
> 125 g (4½ oz) fat-free or light mozzarella cheese, grated
> 30 g (1 oz) freshly grated Parmesan cheese

Preheat the grill. Coat a heavy baking sheet and a 32 × 23-cm (13 × 9-in) glass baking dish with olive oil cooking spray.

In a cup, mix the herb seasoning, salt, red pepper flakes and garlic powder. Arrange the aubergine slices on the prepared baking sheet; mist lightly with olive oil cooking spray and sprinkle with some herb mixture. Turn and repeat on the other side.

Grill 8–13 cm (3–5 in) from the heat, turning once, until lightly browned and very tender, 8–10 minutes. Arrange in a single layer in the prepared baking dish.

Arrange the courgette on the baking sheet. Spray and season as for the aubergine. Grill until tender (it won't really brown), 8–10 minutes. Arrange over the aubergine. Turn the oven to 230°C/450°F/gas 8.

Spoon the sauce over the vegetables, spreading it evenly. Sprinkle evenly with the cheeses. Bake, uncovered, until heated and bubbly, about 10 minutes.

Makes 4 servings

Per serving: 130 calories, 2 g fat, 1 g saturated fat, 13 g protein, 16 g carbohydrates, 2 g dietary fibre, 640 mg sodium

Dining for One

½ teaspoon dried Italian herb seasoning

Pinch salt

Pinch crushed red pepper flakes

Pinch garlic powder

5–9-cm (2–3½-in) lengthwise slices peeled aubergine

5–9-cm (2–3½-in) lengthwise slices courgette

60 ml (2 fl oz) low-fat marinara sauce

30 g (1 oz) light mozzarella cheese, grated

1 tablespoon freshly grated Parmesan cheese

Preheat the grill. Coat a heavy baking sheet and a small baking dish (about 20 × 13 cm/8 × 5 in) with olive oil cooking spray.

In a cup, mix the herb seasoning, salt, red pepper flakes and garlic powder. Arrange the aubergine and courgette on the prepared baking sheet; mist lightly with olive oil cooking spray, and sprinkle with some herb mixture. Turn and repeat on the other side.

Grill 8–13 cm/3–5 in) from the heat, turning once, until very tender, 8–10 minutes. Arrange in the prepared baking dish. Turn the oven to 220°C/425°F/gas 7.

Top the vegetables with the sauce, spreading it evenly; sprinkle with the cheeses. Bake, uncovered, until heated and bubbly, about 10 minutes.

Green and White Dip

Prep: 2 minutes • Cook: 6 minutes

Serve this as a hot main course or spread it on cucumber slices or pepper wedges for an appetizer.

> 150 g (5½ oz) frozen cut-leaf spinach (from a bag)
> 2 tablespoons water
> 125 g (4½ oz) Quark soft cheese
> ¼ teaspoon dried Italian herb seasoning
> Pinch salt
> Pinch garlic powder
> 2 tablespoons grated light mozzarella cheese

In a small, deep, microwave-safe bowl or dish, place the spinach and water. Cover with waxed paper or vented plastic wrap. Microwave on High for 1 minute, until defrosted.

Drain in a sieve, pressing out the excess moisture. Return to the cooking dish.

With a fork, mix in the Quark, herb seasoning, salt and garlic powder. Spread flat in the dish.

Cover with waxed paper or vented plastic wrap and microwave on High for 1½ minutes, until heated and slightly puffed. Sprinkle with the mozzarella and microwave, uncovered, 15 to 30 seconds longer, until the cheese has melted. Let stand a few moments before serving.

Makes 1 serving

Per serving: 150 calories, 5 g fat, 2 g saturated fat, 18 g protein, 9 g carbohydrates, 2 g dietary fibre, 750 mg sodium

Creole Crumbed Prawns

Prep: 10 minutes • Cook: 33 minutes

Don't try to crush the GG Crispbreads in a food processor; it doesn't work too well. Instead, crumble them up with your hands, put them in a resealable plastic freezer bag, and crush with a rolling pin for a super aerobic workout. If the Creole spice blend is unavailable you can make your own: use 2½ tablespoons of sweet paprika, 2 teaspoons each of garlic powder and salt, and 1 teaspoon each of white pepper, black pepper, cayenne, chilli, dried basil and thyme. This will give you enough to make the dish a few times more.

> **4 large egg whites**
> **3 to 4 teaspoons Creole spice blend**
> **2 teaspoons grated lime zest**
> **½–1 teaspoon Tabasco sauce**
> **⅛ teaspoon salt**
> **10 GG Scandinavian Bran Crispbreads, ground to crumbs by hand (see above)**
> **685 g (1½ lb) peeled and deveined large prawns, tails left on**
> **Lime wedges (optional)**

Preheat the oven to 200°C/400°F/gas 6. Coat 2 heavy or nonstick baking sheets with olive oil cooking spray.

In a large bowl, whisk the egg whites until foamy. Beat in the Creole spice blend, lime zest, Tabasco and salt. Place the crispbread crumbs on a plate.

Place the prawns in the egg white mixture and toss to coat. One at a time, roll a prawn in the crumbs, pressing them lightly onto the surface so the crumbs adhere. Arrange the crumbed prawns in single layers on the prepared baking sheets.

Mist the prawns lightly with olive oil cooking spray. Bake until the prawns are just opaque in the thickest part, 16 to 18 minutes.

Serve hot with lime wedges, if you like.

Makes 4 servings

Per serving: 163 calories, 3 g fat, 0.5 g saturated fat, 20 g protein, 17 g carbohydrates, 3 g dietary fibre, 371 mg sodium

Baked Sole with Key West Slaw

Prep: 12 minutes ● Cook: 20 minutes

Normally mild-flavoured, sole gets zing from a Cajun-style mix of spices. If sole is not available, use flounder instead — but remember that thicker fillets will take longer to cook. The slaw can be tossed together a few hours ahead, but it's best eaten the day it's prepared.

For the slaw:

60 ml (2 fl oz) extra-light mayonnaise

½ teaspoon grated lime zest

½ teaspoon grated orange zest

2 tablespoons fresh lime juice

¼ teaspoon coarsely ground black pepper

⅛ teaspoon salt

200 g (7 oz) bagged tricolour slaw mix (cabbage, carrots and red cabbage)

150 g (5½ oz) thin red or yellow pepper strips, each cut in half

2 tablespoons chopped sweet white onion

For the sole:

800 g (1¾ lb) sole fillets, cut in half along the centre seam, bones at top removed

1 tablespoon fresh lime juice

½ teaspoon paprika

½ teaspoon salt

¼ teaspoon dried thyme

Pinch each garlic powder and cayenne pepper

To make the slaw: In a medium bowl, whisk the mayonnaise, lime and orange zests, lime juice, pepper and salt until blended. Add the slaw mix, pepper and onion and mix with a fork. Set aside or cover and refrigerate until ready to serve.

To make the sole: Preheat the oven to 200°C/400°F/gas 6. Coat a rimmed baking sheet with olive oil cooking spray.

Place the sole on the prepared baking sheet, folding the thin ends underneath, and drizzle the fillets with the lime juice. In a cup, mix the paprika, salt, thyme, garlic powder and cayenne. Sprinkle evenly over the sole, spreading it with your fingers.

Bake the sole until it just flakes and is opaque in the thickest part, 10–12 minutes. Transfer the sole to plates, spooning any juices over, and serve with the slaw.

Makes 4 servings

Per serving: 232 calories, 7 g fat, 1 g saturated fat, 35 g protein, 7 g carbohydrates, 2 g dietary fibre, 609 mg sodium

Dr G's Renowned Crab Meat-Stuffed Mushrooms

Prep: 8 minutes • Cook: 23 minutes

I like to serve six to eight of these delightful mushrooms as a light main dish. I also serve a few of them as a first course when entertaining friends.

> **16 large white open-cup mushrooms, stems pulled out**
> **170 g (6 oz) crab meat, picked over**
> **3 tablespoons chopped fresh flat-leaf parsley**
> **3 tablespoons chopped spring onions**
> **3 tablespoons grated fresh Parmesan cheese**
> **1 tablespoon vermouth or dry white wine**
> **1 garlic clove, crushed**
> **⅛ teaspoon freshly ground black pepper**
> **60 g (2 oz) light mozzarella cheese, grated**

Preheat the oven to 190°C/375°F/gas 5. Coat a 32 × 23-cm (13 × 9-in) baking tray with olive oil cooking spray. Arrange the mushrooms open side up in the prepared tray.

In a medium bowl, lightly mix together the crab meat, parsley, spring onions, Parmesan, vermouth or wine, garlic and pepper with a fork.

Stuff the mixture into the mushrooms. Sprinkle with the mozzarella.

Bake until the mushrooms are tender and start to release juices and the cheese has melted, 15–18 minutes. Serve hot.

Makes 16 stuffed mushrooms

Per serving (4 mushrooms): 160 calories, 8 g fat, 4 g saturated fat, 19 g protein, 1 g carbohydrates, 1 g dietary fibre, 371 mg sodium

Grilled Snapper with Orange and Spring Onions

Prep: 7 minutes ● Marinate: 30 minutes ● Cook: 10 minutes

Serve this succulent dish with an assortment of steamed vegetables, perhaps asparagus, green beans and yellow courgette. Any white-fleshed fish will work here: try sea bass, thick sole fillets or halibut. Be sure to sprinkle the spring onions over the fish the moment it comes out of the grill so they'll soften and mellow.

> Four 200 g (7 oz) skinned red snapper fillets
> 1 teaspoon grated orange zest
> 2 tablespoons fresh orange juice
> 1 garlic clove, crushed
> 1½ teaspoons chopped fresh rosemary
> ¼ teaspoon salt
> ⅛ teaspoon freshly ground black pepper
> Pinch crushed red pepper flakes
> 3 tablespoons thinly sliced spring onions

Arrange the fish in a single layer in a shallow dish. In a small bowl, mix the orange zest and juice, garlic, rosemary, salt, black pepper and red pepper flakes. Spoon the mixture evenly over both sides of the fish, spreading it with a spoon. Cover and marinate at cool room temperature or in the refrigerator for 30 minutes.

Preheat the grill. Coat a rimmed baking sheet with olive oil cooking spray.

Transfer the fish to the prepared baking sheet and scrape any remaining marinade onto the fish as well.

Grill 10–15 cm (4–6 in) from the heat until the fish is just opaque in the thickest part, 5–8 minutes. Remove from the heat and immediately sprinkle with the spring onions. Serve.

Makes 4 servings

Per serving: 194 calories, 5 g fat, 0.5 g saturated fat, 36 g protein, 2 g carbohydrates, 0.5 g dietary fibre, 267 mg sodium

Oven-Poached Halibut
with Cucumber and Celery

Prep: 13 minutes • Cook: 30 minutes

You can prepare this soothing dish with any thick, fine-textured white fish, such as cod. The celery and thyme add richness to the poaching stock, without butter or oil. The cucumber is an unusual addition that we think you will enjoy. It's an entirely different vegetable once cooked.

> 350 ml (12 fl oz) fat-free reduced-sodium chicken stock
> 60 ml (2 fl oz) dry vermouth or white wine
> 100 g (3½ oz) thin half-moon slices peeled cucumber
> 100 g (3½ oz) thinly sliced tender celery stalks, with some leaves
> 125 g (4½ oz) thinly sliced leek, well washed
> 2 teaspoons coarsely chopped fresh thyme leaves
> ¼ teaspoon salt
> ¼ teaspoon freshly ground black pepper
> 800 g (1¾ lb) skinned halibut fillet, cut in 8 equal pieces

Preheat the oven to 220°C/425°F/gas 7. Set out a large, deep ovenproof frying pan (wrap handle with heavy-duty foil if it is not ovenproof).

In the pan, stir together the stock, vermouth or wine, cucumber, celery, leek, 1 teaspoon thyme and ⅛ teaspoon each salt and pepper. Bring to the boil over high heat. Reduce the heat to medium-low, cover, and simmer until the vegetables are tender, about 10 minutes.

Meanwhile, season the halibut with the remaining 1 teaspoon thyme and remaining ⅛ teaspoon each salt and pepper.

Arrange the halibut in a single layer over the vegetables in the pan. Bring to a low simmer. Cover with foil or a lid and place in the oven. Bake until just opaque in the thickest part, 12–14 minutes, depending on thickness.

Serve the halibut with the vegetables and pan juices in heated soup plates.

Makes 4 servings

Per serving: 208 calories, 5 g fat, 1 g saturated fat, 36 g protein, 2 g carbohydrates, 1 g dietary fibre, 350 mg sodium

Oven-Steamed Salmon, Hong Kong-Style

Prep: 8 minutes ● Cook: 22 minutes

This delicious and very calorie-wise preparation is also wonderful with scallops or prawns. And it's so versatile that you can prepare it for just one serving; see Dining for One version on the opposite page for cooking times and amounts. If you like, sprinkle each portion with ¼ teaspoon of toasted sesame seeds before serving.

> 3 tablespoons reduced-sodium soy sauce
>
> 2 large garlic cloves, crushed
>
> 1 tablespoon finely chopped peeled fresh ginger
>
> 1 tablespoon medium dry sherry
>
> 685 g (1½ lb) skinned salmon fillet, cut into four 170 g (6 oz) portions
>
> ⅛ teaspoon salt
>
> 1 bunch spring onions, diagonally sliced

Preheat oven to 220°C/425°F/gas 7. Set out two rimmed baking sheets.

In a cup, mix the soy sauce, garlic, ginger and sherry. Tear off four 45-cm (18-in) long pieces of heavy-duty foil. Fold each piece of foil crosswise like a book, then open up. Coat one half of each sheet with olive oil cooking spray. In the centre of the sprayed half, place a piece of salmon and sprinkle with some salt. Spoon 1 heaped tablespoon of the soy sauce mixture over each piece of salmon and sprinkle with ¼ of the spring onions.

Fold the other side of the foil over the food. Crimp the edges tightly to seal. Place the packets on the baking sheets. Bake until the salmon is just opaque in the thickest part, about 20 minutes. Slide the contents of the packets onto warmed dinner plates and serve right away.

Makes 4 servings

Per serving: 330 calories, 20 g fat, 4 g saturated fat, 33 g protein, 2 g carbohydrates, 1 g dietary fibre, 554 mg sodium

Scallop Variation
Prepare as directed above, using 685 g (1½ lb) sea scallops (tough tendons at sides removed), rinsed and patted dry. Bake for 15 minutes, or until just opaque in the thickest part.

Prawn Variation
Prepare as directed above, using 685 g (1½ lb) peeled and deveined large prawns. Bake for 15 minutes, or until just opaque in the thickest part.

Dining for One
> 2 teaspoons reduced-sodium soy sauce
> 1 medium garlic clove, crushed
> ¾ teaspoon finely chopped peeled fresh ginger
> ¾ teaspoon medium dry sherry
> One 170 g (6 oz) skinned salmon fillet, 170 g (6 oz) peeled and deveined prawns, or 170 g (6 oz) scallops, tough tendons at sides removed, rinsed and patted dry
> Pinch salt
> 30 g (1 oz) diagonally sliced spring onions

Prepare as directed above, using these amounts. Bake for 15 minutes, or until just opaque in the thickest part.

Seafood in Brodo

Prep: 25 minutes ● Cook: 25 minutes

In Italian, *brodo* means watery soup or stock. Here seafood is simmered in a richly flavoured stock, giving it succulence without adding fat. Vary the seafood depending on your taste and what looks good at the fish counter. You can make this with all scallops, if that strikes your fancy, or swap clams for mussels – they'll cook in about the same amount of time. For instructions on cleaning mussels, see page 251.

> 480 ml (16 fl oz) fat-free reduced-sodium chicken stock
>
> 1 small onion, halved and thinly sliced
>
> 3 tablespoons dry white wine
>
> 1 tablespoon white rice wine vinegar
>
> 3 garlic cloves, thinly sliced
>
> 1 sprig fresh thyme or $\frac{1}{8}$ teaspoon dried
>
> 1 small to medium courgette, sliced into thin half-moons
>
> 1 medium red pepper, cut into thin strips, strips cut in half
>
> 170 g (6 oz) peeled and deveined large prawns, tails left on
>
> 170 g (6 oz) scallops, rinsed and patted dry, cut in half through
>   the centre, tough tendon at sides removed
>
> 12 medium mussels, well scrubbed and debearded
>
> 1 medium plum tomato, diced
>
> 3 tablespoons chopped flat-leaf parsley

In a wide saucepan or large deep frying pan, stir the stock, onion, wine, vinegar, garlic and thyme. Bring to a boil over high heat. Reduce the heat to medium, cover, and simmer for 5 minutes.

Add the courgette and pepper; cover and simmer until tender, about 5 minutes longer. Stir in the prawns, scallops and mussels. Cover and cook, stirring occasionally, until the prawns and scallops are just opaque in the thickest part and the mussels have opened, 4–6 minutes.

Remove from the heat and stir in the tomato and parsley. Serve immediately in deep bowls.

Makes 4 servings

Per serving: 130 calories, 2 g fat, 0.5 g saturated fat, 19 g protein, 7 g carbohydrates, 2 g dietary fibre, 476 mg sodium

Roasted Sage-Lemon Salmon

Prep: 4 minutes ● Cook: 14 minutes

Sage – often thought of as the main flavouring in turkey stuffing – has a natural affinity for salmon. This is a super recipe that goes together in minutes. Any leftovers are terrific cold for lunch the next day or can be used to prepare Grilled Salmon Salad (page 234).

> 570 g (1¼ lb) skinned salmon fillet, cut in four 140 g (5 oz)
>   portions
> 2 tablespoon fresh lemon juice
> 1 teaspoon dried sage, crumbled
> ¾ teaspoon coarsely ground black pepper
> ½ teaspoon sea salt
> Lemon wedges

Preheat the oven to 230°C/450°F/gas 8. Coat a rimmed baking sheet with olive oil cooking spray.

Place the salmon on the prepared baking sheet. Drizzle evenly with the lemon juice. In a cup, mix the sage, pepper and salt with your fingers. Sprinkle evenly over the salmon.

Roast the salmon until just opaque in the thickest part, 9–12 minutes, depending on thickness. Transfer to warmed dinner plates and serve with lemon wedges.

Makes 4 servings

Per serving: 260 calories, 17 g fat, 3 g saturated fat, 26 g protein, 1 g carbohydrates, 0 g dietary fibre, 431 mg sodium

Seafood Salad Positano

Prep: 20 minutes ● Cook: 15 minutes ● Standing: 15 minutes or longer

Elegant for a summer dinner in the garden or at the seaside, this is also good cold the next day. It's perfect for company. Serve with steamed asparagus.

240 ml (8 fl oz) fat-free reduced-sodium chicken stock

80 ml (3 fl oz) dry white wine

2 garlic cloves, crushed

¼ teaspoon salt

⅛–¼ teaspoon crushed red pepper flakes

285 g (10 oz) peeled and deveined large prawns, tails left on

285 g (10 oz) scallops, rinsed and patted dry, tough tendons at sides removed, cut in half crosswise

115 g (4 oz) skinned firm white fish fillet, such as monkfish or halibut, cut in 2.5-cm (1-in) chunks

115 g (4 oz) crab meat, picked over

60 g (2 oz) thinly sliced tender celery hearts

90 g (3 oz) quartered water-packed canned artichoke hearts, drained

30 g (1 oz) chopped flat-leaf parsley

60 g (2 oz) sliced water-packed jarred roasted red peppers, drained

3 tablespoons chopped pitted kalamata olives

2 tablespoons fresh lemon juice

In a large deep frying pan, bring the stock, wine, garlic, ⅛ teaspoon salt and red pepper flakes to the boil over high heat. Reduce the heat to medium, cover, and simmer for 5 minutes to blend the flavours.

Stir in the prawns, scallops and fish. Cover and cook, gently stirring often, until the seafood is opaque in the thickest part, 4–5 minutes.

Remove from the heat. With a slotted spoon, gently transfer the seafood to a salad bowl, reserving 60 ml (2 fl oz) of the cooking liquid. Cover loosely and let cool to lukewarm, about 15 minutes.

Gently fold in the crab meat, celery, artichoke hearts, parsley, peppers, olives, lemon juice, the reserved cooking liquid and remaining ⅛ teaspoon salt. Serve immediately or cover and chill to serve later.

Makes 4 servings

Per serving: 203 calories, 6 g fat, 1 g saturated fat, 31 g protein, 4 g carbohydrates, 2 g dietary fibre, 1130 mg sodium

Mussels with Soy and Sherry

Prep: 20 minutes ● Cook: 24 minutes

To clean the mussels, scrub them under cold running water using a stiff brush. Discard any with broken shells or mussels that are open and don't close up when tapped or pressed shut. Pull out the 'beard' if it's there; it will be sticking out along the unhinged side. Rinse the mussels again.

> 240 ml (8 fl oz) fat-free reduced-sodium chicken stock
> 60 ml (2 fl oz) medium dry sherry
> 3 garlic cloves, crushed
> 1 tablespoon finely chopped peeled fresh ginger
> 1 bunch spring onions, thinly sliced
> 2 tablespoons reduced-sodium soy sauce
> 48 medium mussels (about 1.4 kg/3 lb), scrubbed and debearded (see above)

In a wide saucepan or large deep frying pan, stir together the stock, sherry, garlic and ginger. Bring to a boil over high heat.

Reduce the heat to medium, cover, and simmer for 3 minutes. Stir in the spring onions and soy sauce; cover and simmer 2 minutes longer.

Add the mussels; stir gently and increase the heat to high. Cover and cook the mussels, shaking the pot and stirring frequently, until the shells are open, about 5 minutes. Remove from the heat and discard any unopened shells. Spoon the mussels into soup plates, ladling the cooking juices over them. Serve right away.

Makes 4 servings

Per serving: 123 calories, 2 g fat, 0.5 g saturated fat, 20 g protein, 2 g carbohydrates, 0.5 g dietary fibre, 490 mg sodium

Scallop and Vegetable Packets

Prep: 12 minutes • Cook: 20 minutes

This is a great dish for busy people. In no time at all the fish and veggies are on the table – with no stirring and no pots to wash! Make this for the family or just for yourself (see Dining for One version on the opposite page).

> 75 g (2½ oz) baby spinach
> 230 g (8 oz) sliced yellow courgette
> 455 g (1 lb) scallops, rinsed and patted dry, tough tendons at
>   sides removed
> 20 slender asparagus spears, tough ends snapped off, cut in 5-cm
>   (2-in) lengths
> 4 slices sweet onion, rings separated
> 4 slices tomato
> 30 g (1 oz) chopped flat-leaf parsley
> 4 teaspoons vermouth or dry white wine
> ½ teaspoon salt
> ¼ teaspoon freshly ground black pepper

Preheat the oven to 220°C/425°F/gas 7. Set out two baking sheets.

Tear off four 50-cm (20-in) long sheets of heavy-duty foil. Fold each piece of foil crosswise like a book, then open up. Coat one half of each sheet with olive oil cooking spray.

In the centre of each sprayed half, arrange a quarter of the spinach, courgette, scallops, asparagus, onion and tomato. Sprinkle with a heaped tablespoon parsley. Drizzle with 1 teaspoon vermouth or wine and sprinkle with some salt and pepper.

Fold the other side of the foil over the food. Crimp the edges tightly to seal. Place the packets on the baking sheets.

Bake until the scallops are opaque in the thickest part and the vegetables are tender, about 20 minutes.

Transfer the contents of each packet to a heated dinner plate and serve right away.

Makes 4 servings

Per serving: 156 calories, 4 g fat, 1 g saturated fat, 25 g protein, 5 g carbohydrates, 4 g dietary fibre, 562 mg sodium

Dining for One

    20 g (¾ oz) spinach

    60 g (2 oz) sliced yellow courgette

    115 g (4 oz) scallops

    5 slender asparagus spears, tough ends snapped off, cut in 5-cm
       (2-in) lengths

    1 slice sweet onion, rings separated

    1 slice tomato

    1 heaped tablespoon chopped flat-leaf parsley

    1 teaspoon vermouth or dry white wine

    ⅛ teaspoon salt

    Pinch freshly ground black pepper

Prepare as previously directed. Bake until the scallops are opaque in the thickest part and the vegetables are tender, about 20 minutes.

Yucatan-Style Grilled Swordfish

Prep: 6 minutes ● Marinate: 15 minutes ● Cook: 14 minutes

To provide deep flavour, lime zest, garlic and aromatic spices are smashed to a paste and spread over the fish before grilling. We loved the fish atop tender baby greens, letting the juices dress and wilt them – adding a spritz of lime juice.

Note: Swordfish is often sold with the skin on, but the skin is tough and unpleasant and should be removed. Ask the fishmonger to do this, or do it yourself with a sharp knife. Also trim off the dark reddish portions, which can be bitter. Then cut the fish into 200-g (7-oz) portions. You'll need to purchase a somewhat heavier piece than you need to account for the trimming.

> 1 tablespoon grated lime zest
> 2 large garlic cloves, coarsely chopped
> $1\frac{3}{4}$ teaspoons chilli powder
> $\frac{1}{2}$ teaspoon ground cumin
> $\frac{1}{2}$ teaspoon sea salt
> Pinch ground cinnamon
> 3 tablespoons fresh lime juice
> 800 g ($1\frac{3}{4}$ lb) 2.5-cm (1-in) thick trimmed swordfish steaks (see note), cut in four 200 g (7 oz) portions
> Lime wedges

On a cutting board, finely chop the lime zest and garlic together. Mix in the chilli powder, cumin, salt and cinnamon. Using the flat side of a chef's knife, rub the mixture on the board to form a slightly damp paste. Scrape into a cup and stir in the lime juice.

Put the swordfish on a large plate. Spoon the paste over both sides, spreading it with the back of a spoon. Cover and let stand for 15 minutes.

Meanwhile, place the oven rack as close to the grill element as possible and preheat the grill. Coat a grill-pan rack with olive oil cooking spray.

Place the swordfish on the prepared grill pan; scrape any paste from the plate on top. Grill until just opaque in the thickest part, 5–7 minutes.

Serve hot with lime wedges.

Serves 4

Per serving: 190 calories, 5 g fat, 0.5 g saturated fat, 36 g protein, 1 g carbohydrates, 0.5 g dietary fibre, 481 mg sodium

Strawberry Soup

Prep: 10 minutes

This refreshing dessert is best freshly made.

> **455 g (1 lb) fresh strawberries, rinsed and hulled**
> **75 g (2½ oz) low-carb strawberry preserve**
> **200 g (7 oz) natural fat-free yogurt**
> **Pinch ground cinnamon**

Thinly slice about 200 g (7 oz) strawberries and reserve. Cut the rest into thick slices.

In a food processor, process the thick-sliced strawberries and preserve until finely puréed. Add the yogurt and process until smooth.

Transfer to a bowl and stir in the reserved sliced strawberries and cinnamon. Ladle into bowls or mugs and serve.

Makes 4 servings

Per serving: 82 calories, 1 g fat, 0 g saturated fat, 4 g protein, 16 g carbohydrates, 1.5 g dietary fibre, 52 mg sodium

Lime-Garlic Grilled Poussins

**Prep: 10 minutes • Marinate: at least 2 hours or overnight •
Cook: 40 minutes**

If you like spicy, use ½ teaspoon crushed red pepper flakes or add a crushed chilli to the marinade. For deepest flavour, marinate the birds overnight.

> **2 poussins, each about 570g (1¼ lb)**
> **80 ml (3 fl oz) fresh lime juice**
> **3 garlic cloves, crushed**
> **1½ tablespoons reduced-sodium soy sauce**
> **2 teaspoons grated orange zest**
> **¼ teaspoon crushed red pepper flakes**

Cut the wing tips off the birds. With poultry shears, cut down along both sides of the bird's backbone to remove it and discard. Open the bird up and cut it in half down the centre of the breast. Repeat with the other poussin.

In a measuring cup, stir together the lime juice, garlic, soy sauce, orange zest and red pepper flakes. Put the birds in a resealable plastic freezer bag; pour in the marinade. Seal the bag and squish it so the marinade coats evenly. Place the bag in a bowl in case of leaks. Marinate the birds in the refrigerator at least 2 hours or overnight.

Heat a barbecue grill to medium. Oil the grill.

Remove the birds from the marinade. Drain the marinade into a small saucepan, bring to a full boil and boil for 2 minutes.

Place the birds skin side down on the grill. Baste with some marinade. Grill until lightly browned on the underside, about 10 minutes. Use a metal spatula to loosen the birds and turn.

Continue grilling, basting occasionally, and turning and moving as necessary, until no longer pink in the thickest part, 15–20 minutes longer. Discard any remaining marinade. Serve the birds, removing the skin before eating.

Makes 4 servings

Per serving: 390 calories, 16 g fat, 6 g saturated fat, 50 g protein, 1 g carbohydrates, 0 g dietary fibre, 346 mg sodium

Micro-Spice Butternut Squash

Prep: 3 minutes ● Cook: 7 minutes

For this recipe, buy a small butternut squash and, using a sturdy vegetable peeler, cut and peel what you need. This would be nice topped with a tablespoon of fat-free natural yogurt. I find that this dish makes a nice complement to fish.

> 145 g (5 oz) peeled and seeded butternut squash cut into 2.5-cm (1-in) chunks
>
> 2 tablespoons water
>
> ⅛ teaspoon ground cinnamon
>
> Pinch ground nutmeg
>
> Pinch salt
>
> Pinch freshly ground black pepper

Put the squash chunks in a shallow microwave-safe dish or pie dish. Drizzle with the water and sprinkle with the cinnamon, nutmeg, salt and pepper. Toss to mix.

Cover with waxed paper or vented plastic wrap and microwave on High until the squash is tender, 5–6 minutes. Let stand a few minutes before serving, as the squash will be very hot.

Makes 1 serving

Per serving: 30 calories, 0.5 g fat, 0 g saturated fat, 1 g protein, 4 g carbohydrates, 1.5 g dietary fibre, 389 mg sodium

A LAST WORD ON MAINTENANCE

The strategies and guidelines that have helped you lose weight apply even more on maintenance because your body is lighter and needs fewer calories than when you started. During maintenance, thinking historically, not just calorically, remains critical. As I've said throughout this book, the same people gain back the same weight on the same foods again and again. Just because you've lost weight and changed your size doesn't mean you've lost your vulnerability or changed your history with problem foods. *If at any time you find that introducing a certain food(s) stimulates cravings and overconsumption, or you find that your appetite increases after you eat that food, eliminate it!*

I encourage you to read and reread the guidelines and protective strategies in the Tenth Commandment, Losing Weight Is Half the Job; Keeping It Off Is the Other Half. Complacency is the enemy of thin. You can eat the right foods, but if you don't practise the right behaviours, you'll just be another dieter who loses weight only to gain it back. To help protect you against this disappointment, I created the Maintenance New Scale as an early warning system. Weigh yourself daily or several times a week, and weigh your behaviour and thinking weekly on the Maintenance New Scale. Truly, behaviour predicts the direction your bathroom scales will be heading. That's why the Maintenance New Scale is such a unique and powerful tool in my work.

'How many calories can I add on maintenance?' is a question I'm frequently asked by clients who are close to their goal weight. If you're losing less than a half a kilogram or a pound a week, your body is probably telling you there's little room in your calorie budget for additions. At most, you may be looking to add an extra 500 calories a week. If your weight loss has stopped before or as you approach the goal and you still want to add new foods, you may do so one or two times a week. You may find that the day after you eat these foods, your weight is up. If it remains up for several days, return to the foods in the 10-day diet until it drops to a lower number. Then you can add a new food or meal. It's like balancing your budget; if you overspend your calorie budget one day, you balance out the excess by returning to the 10-day diet.

Maintenance Food Guidelines

Avoid all foods you have a history of abusing and that you have Boxed Out. Remember to limit the frequency and quantity of foods you have Boxed In – you have lost weight, not your vulnerability to these foods.

Food	Women	Men
Alcohol (excluding drinks that include fruit juice, tonic water, or regular soda)	Occasional use; no more than 1 time a day suggested maximum	Occasional use; no more than 2 times a day suggested maximum
Bagels (I suggest an English muffin)	For occasional use (once a week, preferably on weekends) or avoid	For occasional use (twice a week, preferably on weekends) or avoid
Breakfast cereal (including oatmeal)	A single, measured serving of a high-fibre cereal that contains no added sugar (must be less than 5g of sugar and more than 5g of fibre), 1–5 times a week	Same instruction as for women, but every day is acceptable
Butter and margarine	Avoid butter, or use no more than 1 tsp. Avoid margarines with hydrogenated or partially hydrogenated oil. If margarine is used in lieu of oil, limit to 1–2 times a day	Same instructions as for women, but 3–4 times a day
Confectionery	To be used infrequently or on special occasions; best to choose low-calorie options	Same instructions as for women
Desserts	For occasional use or avoid. If you want to have desserts more frequently, choose something from the 10-day diet, or a Weight Watchers dessert	For occasional use or avoid. Same instruction as for women

Food	Women	Men
French fries	Avoid or for occasional use only	Avoid or for occasional use only
Fruits (except grapes, cherries, or cut-up fruit)	2–3 a day	3–4 a day
Fruit juice (in lieu of a serving of fruit)	120–180 ml (4–6 fl oz) a day	180–240 ml (6–8 fl oz) a day
Full-calorie gourmet meals	1–2 a week	3–4 a week
Olive oil or similar vegetable oil	1–2 tbsp a day	2–3 tbsp a day
Pasta (counts as a full-calorie gourmet meal)	Avoid pasta made with cheese or oil; maximum of 115 g (4 oz) once a week, or a 60 g (2 oz) appetizer twice a week	Avoid pasta made with cheese or oil; max. of 145 g (5 oz) once a week, or a 60–90 g (2–3 oz) appetizer twice a week
Pizza (counts as a gourmet meal)	Only choose a cheese or vegetable topping; 1 slice a week	Only choose a cheese or vegetable topping; 2 slices a week
Potato or grains	1 medium potato (preferably boiled) or 75 g (2½ oz) grains, 1–3 times a week	1 medium potato or 115 g (4 oz) of grains, 2–7 times a week
Salad dressings	Prepare with 1 tbsp of olive oil	Prepare with 1–2 tbsp of olive oil
Sandwiches	Occasional use or prepare with 2 slices of light bread or GG Crispbreads	Occasional use or prepare with 2 slices of light bread or GG Crispbreads
Tomato sauce (without oil)	Use as needed	Use as needed

Index

Underscored page references indicate boxed text.

OTHER RODALE BOOKS
AVAILABLE FROM PAN MACMILLAN

1-4050-2101-2	8 Minutes in the Morning	*Jorge Cruise*	£12.99
1-4050-3284-7	Anti-Ageing Prescriptions	*Dr James A. Duke*	£14.99
1-4050-4099-8	Before the Heart Attacks	*Dr H. Robert Superko*	£12.99
1-4050-4179-X	Fit Not Fat at 40+	*The Editors of* Prevention	£12.99
1-4050-3335-5	Picture Perfect Weight Loss	*Dr Howard Shapiro*	£14.99
1-4050-6717-9	The South Beach Diet Cookbook	*Dr Arthur Agatston*	£20
1-4050-3286-3	Stay Fertile Longer	*Mary Kittel*	£12.99
1-4050-3340-1	When Your Body Gets the Blues	*Marie-Annette Brown and Jo Robinson*	£10.99
1-4050-7330-1	The Women's Health Bible	*The Editors of* Prevention	£14.99

All Pan Macmillan titles can be ordered from our website, www.panmacmillan.com, or from your local bookshop and are also available by post from:

Bookpost, PO Box 29, Douglas, Isle of Man IM99 1BQ
Tel: 01624 677237; fax: 01624 670923; e-mail: bookshop@enterprise.net; or visit: www.bookpost.co.uk. Credit cards accepted. Free postage and packing in the United Kingdom

Prices shown above were correct at time of going to press.

Pan Macmillan reserve the right to show new retail prices on covers which may differ from those previously advertised in the text or elsewhere.

For information about buying Rodale titles in **Australia**, contact Pan Macmillan Australia. Tel: 1300 135 113; fax: 1300 135 103; e-mail: customer.service@macmillan.com.au; or visit: www.panmacmillan.com.au

For information about buying Rodale titles in **New Zealand**, contact Macmillan Publishers New Zealand Limited. Tel: (09) 414 0356; fax: (09) 414 0352; e-mail: lyn@macmillan.co.nz; or visit: www.macmillan.co.nz

For information about buying Rodale titles in **South Africa**, contact Pan Macmillan South Africa. Tel: (011) 325 5220; fax: (011) 325 5225; e-mail: roshni@panmacmillan.co.za

RODALE

MACMILLAN